# Colloid Science in Pharmaceutical Nanotechnology

*Edited by Selcan Karakuş*

Published in London, United Kingdom

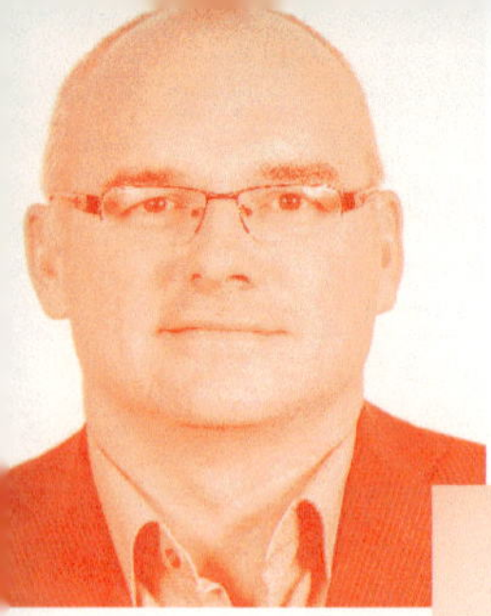
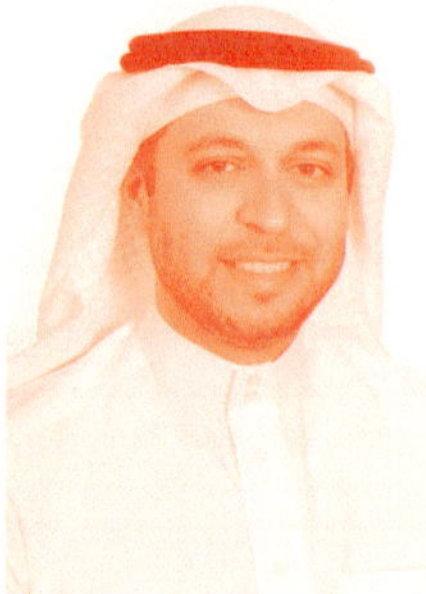
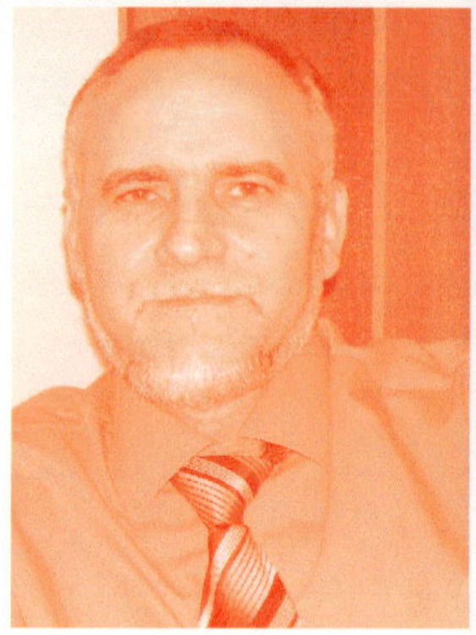
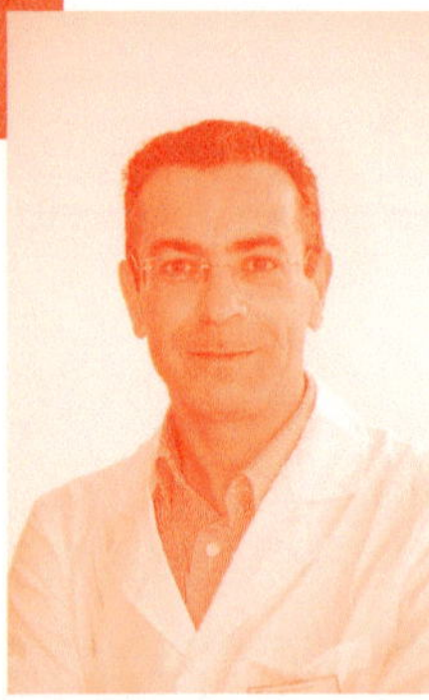
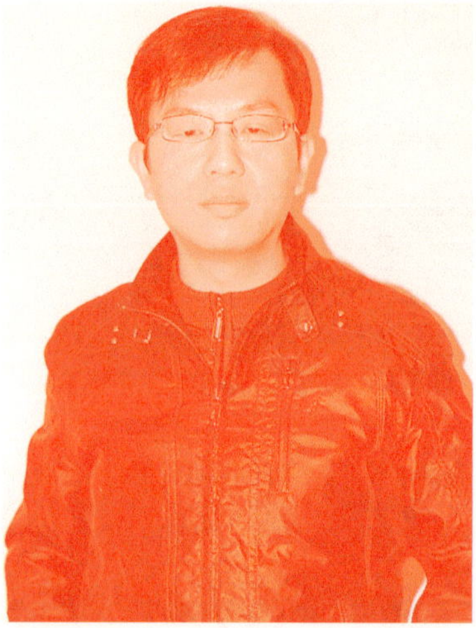
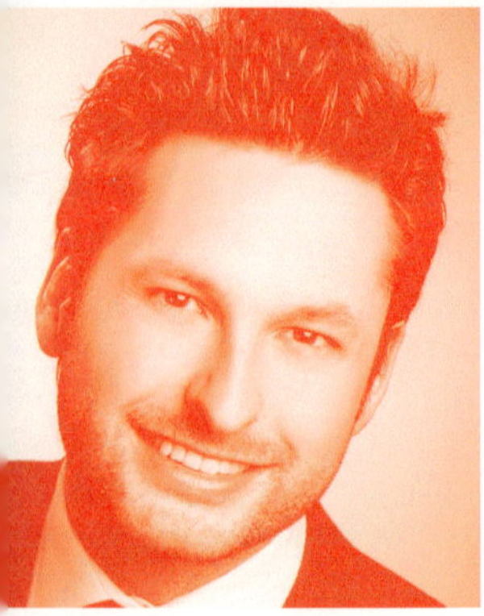
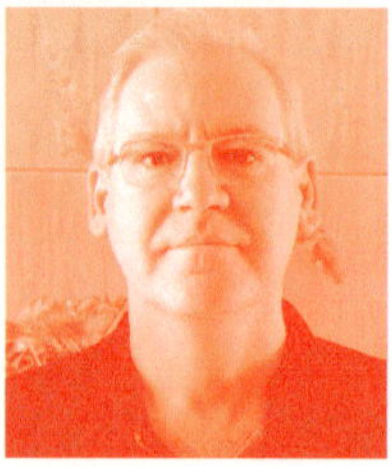

IntechOpen

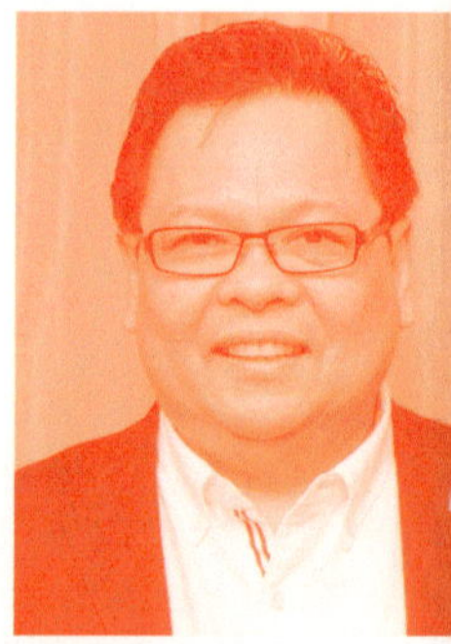
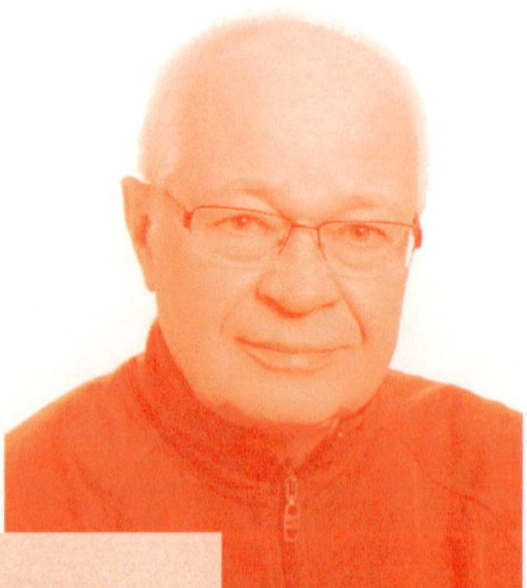
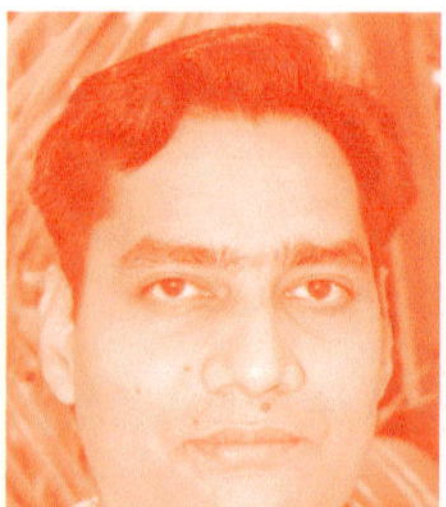
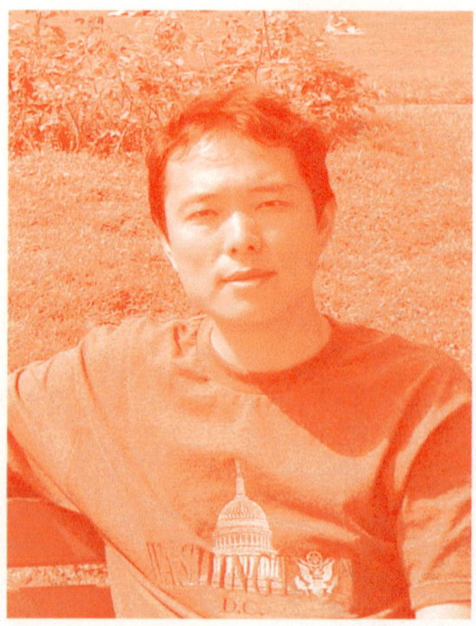
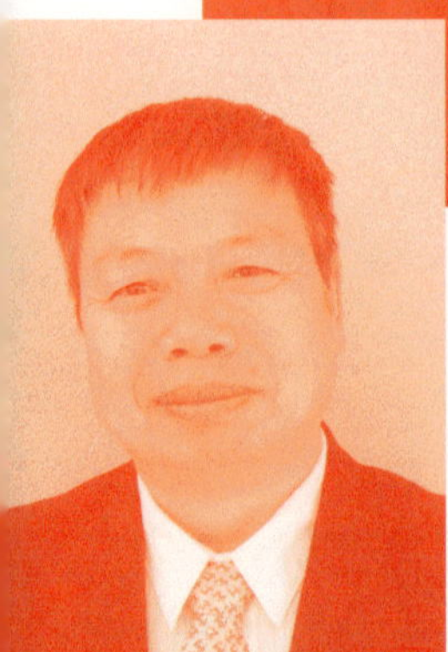
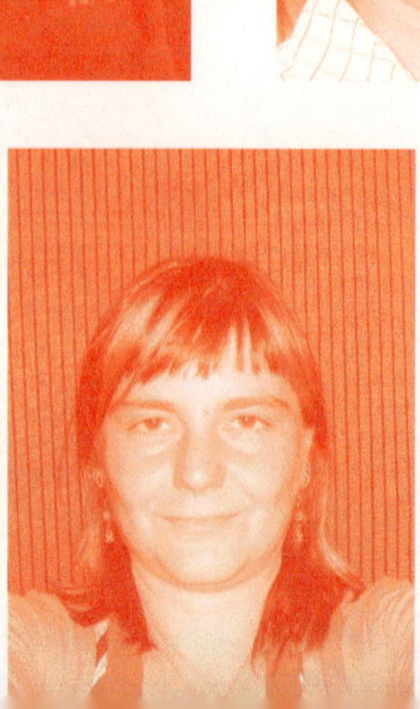

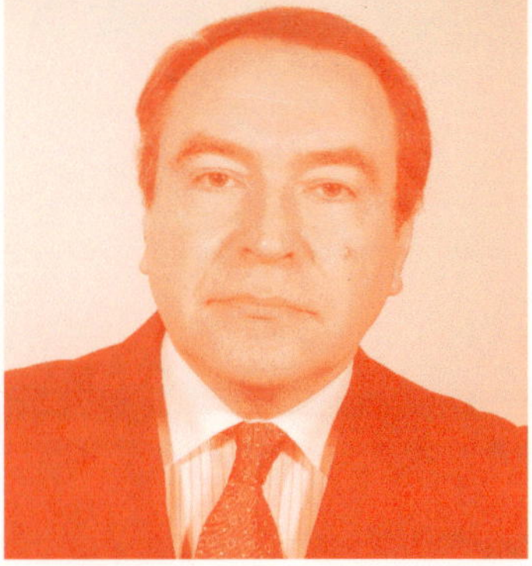
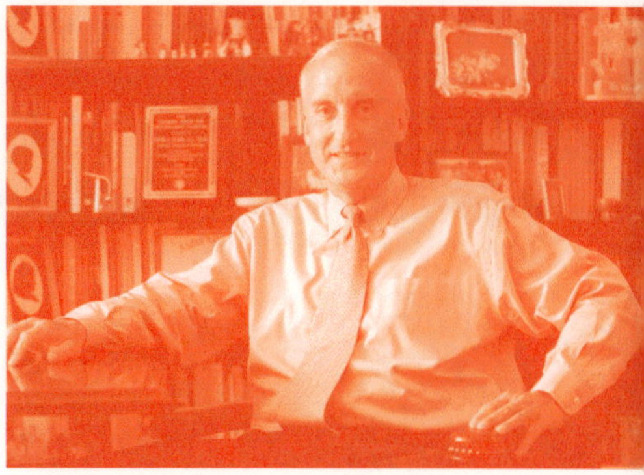
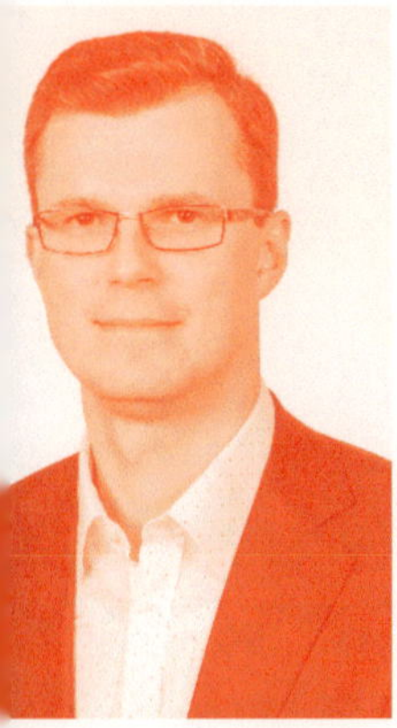
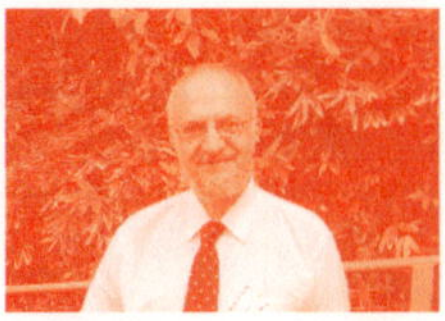
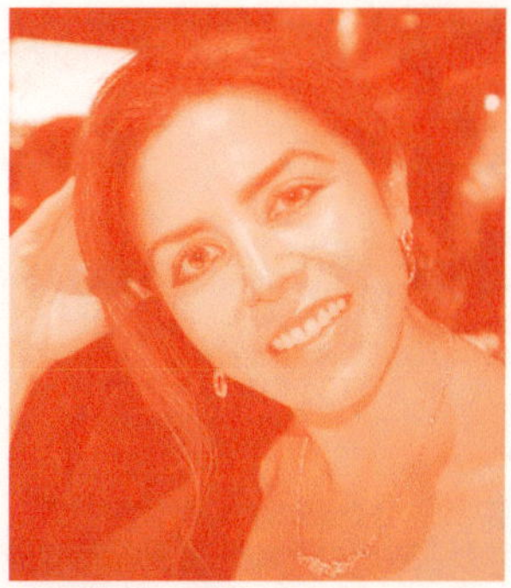

*Supporting open minds since 2005*

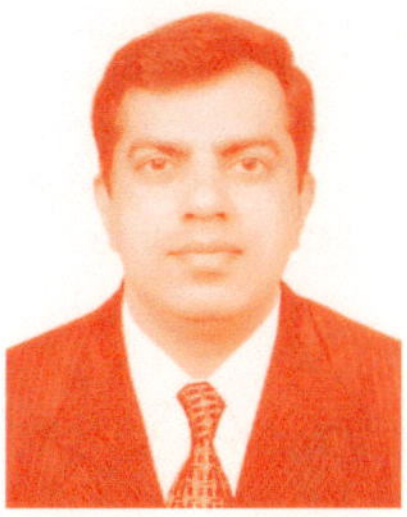
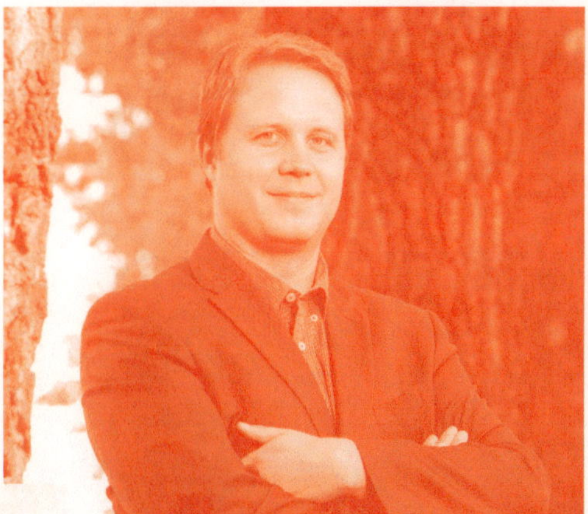
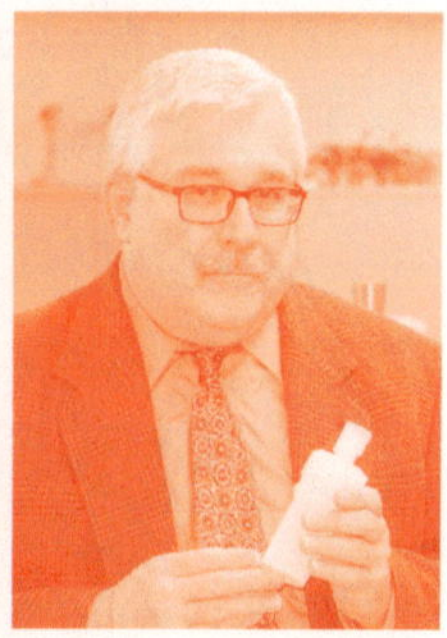
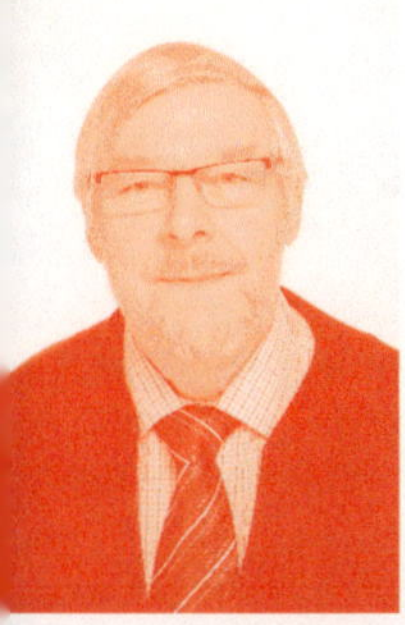
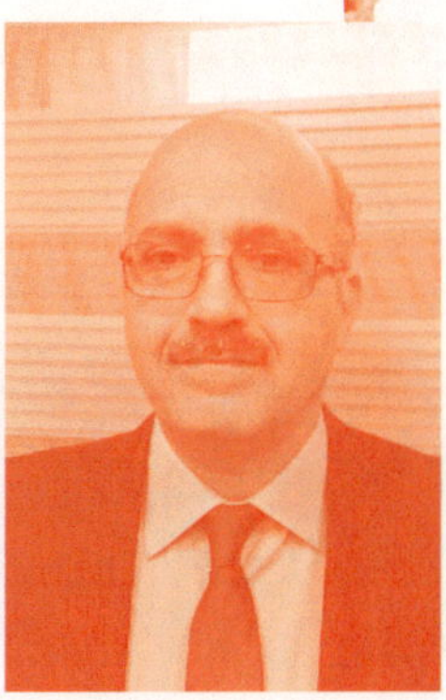
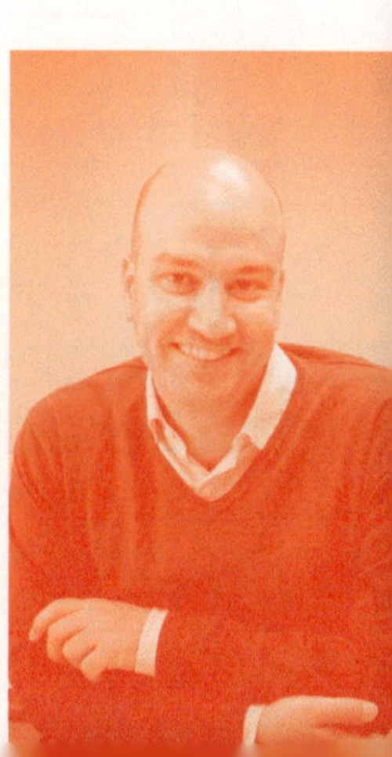
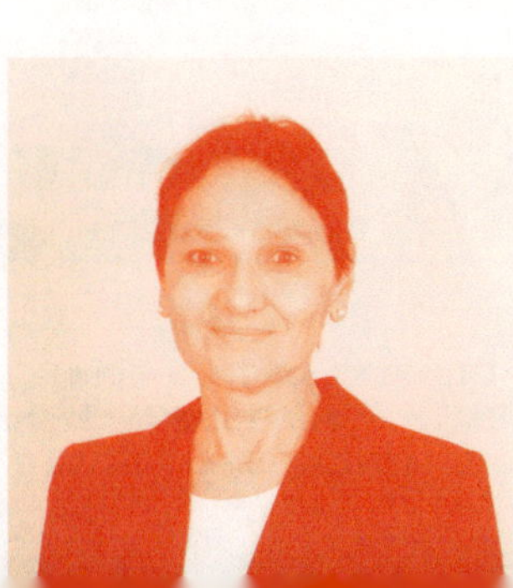

Colloid Science in Pharmaceutical Nanotechnology
http://dx.doi.org/10.5772/intechopen.77406
Edited by Selcan Karakuş

Contributors
Anuj G. Agrawal, Mansi Shah, Rekha Rao, Sunil Kumar, Pooja Lamba, Camillo La Mesa, Gianfranco Risuleo, Haroon Khalid Syed, Tauqeer Mallhi, Mehreen Bashir, Sajid Asghar, Ikram Ullah Khan, Erandi Munasinghe, Maheshi Athapaththu, Lakmal Jayarathne, Lakmal Jayarathna, Rohan Weerasooriya, Athula Bandara, Nelum Karunathilake, Selcan Karakuş, Merve Ilgar, Ezgi Tan, Yeşim Müge Sahin, Nevin Tasaltin, Ayben Kilislioglu



First published in London, United Kingdom, 2020 by IntechOpen
IntechOpen is the global imprint of INTECHOPEN LIMITED, registered in England and Wales, registration number: 11086078, 7th floor, 10 Lower Thames Street, London, EC3R 6AF, United Kingdom
Printed in Croatia

British Library Cataloguing-in-Publication Data
A catalogue record for this book is available from the British Library

Additional hard and PDF copies can be obtained from orders@intechopen.com

Colloid Science in Pharmaceutical Nanotechnology
Edited by Selcan Karakuş
p. cm.
Print ISBN 978-1-78985-595-1
Online ISBN 978-1-78985-596-8
eBook (PDF) ISBN 978-1-83880-498-5

For EU product safety concerns:
IN TECH d.o.o., Prolaz Marije Krucifikse Kozulić 3, 51000 Rijeka, Croatia, info@intechopen.com or visit our website at intechopen.com.

# Meet the editor

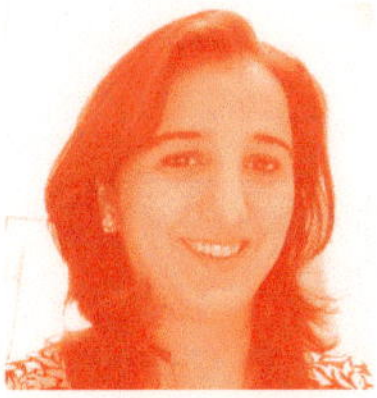

Assistant professor Selcan Karakuş is currently working in the Department of Chemistry, Istanbul University-Cerrahpasa (IUC), Turkey. She received her Master of Science degree in Physical Chemistry from Istanbul University (IU) in 2006 and her Doctor of Philosophy degree in Physical Chemistry from IU in 2011. She has worked as a visiting researcher at the University of Massachusetts, Department of Polymer Science and Engineering and has research experience in drug carrier systems, nanoparticles, nanocomposites, nanoemulsions, self-assembled polymeric nanostructures, and copolymer blends. She has worked on different projects funded by IUC, and has published several research articles and a book chapter on the above fields.

# Contents

# Preface

The definition of a colloidal particle is a micro/nanometer-sized solid particle uniformly dispersed in a solution. In colloidal dispersions, there are two phase systems: continuous phase and dispersed phase (ranging from 1 nm to 1 μm). The colloidal particle/nanoparticle is produced by considering various key factors such as particle size, distribution, polarity, and surface properties. The stability of colloidal dispersion has a role in homogeneous distribution with steric and electrostatic modifications.

Recently, colloidal and nanotechnological approaches have been considered as advanced technologies. Nanotechnology is known as scientific and engineering knowledge that makes it possible to use nanosized materials in special applications. Nanotechnology has developed science and technology by producing superior products and it has a multidisciplinary approach. Nanotechnological products have attracted much attention with many new studies concentrating on colloids and nanoparticles in biotechnology for biomedical and environmental applications. Materials science, engineering, medicine, dentistry, drug delivery, etc. have all used this approach. Knowledge of nanoscience and nanoengineering is being used to produce nanotechnology-based products such as nanoparticles, nanolayers, nanocomposites, nanofibers, oil-in-water nanoemulsions, cyclodextrin-nanosponges, etc. Colloidal particles/nanoparticles are preferred because of their biocompatibility and performance in pharmaceutical applications. For this purpose, colloidal particles are also widely used in the development of novel drug delivery systems for use in diagnosis and treatment.

*Colloid Science in Pharmaceutical Nanotechnology* is comprised of seven chapters that provide an overview of colloidal particle and nanoparticle systems, their physicochemical properties, and pharmaceutical applications. Some of the topics covered are nanoparticle-based drug design, the miscibility of colloidal particles, and the stability of nanoparticles. The preparation and characterization of colloidal systems are discussed in detail. In this book, the authors focus on recent studies, applications, and new technological developments of the fundamental properties of colloidal particle systems. Readers will be able to access recent studies, applications, and new technological developments on colloidal systems. We sincerely thank our authors who have contributed with experience and knowledge to this book. Especially, our thanks go to Erbil Karakuş, Emir Ersel Karakuş and the editorial team from IntechOpen for their assistance in preparing this book.

**Selcan Karakuş**
Assistant Professor,
Department of Chemistry,
Faculty of Engineering,
Istanbul, Turkey

University-Cerrahpasa,
Istanbul, Turkey

# Section 1

# Colloid Science and Nanoparticles

Chapter 1

# The Viscosity Behaviour of PEGylated Locust Bean Gum/Rosin Ester Polymeric Nanoparticles

*Selcan Karakus, Merve Ilgar, Ezgi Tan, Yeşim Müge Sahin, Nevin Tasaltin and Ayben Kilislioglu*

## Abstract

In this study, PEGylated locust bean gum–rosin glycerol ester polymeric nanoparticles (PEG-LBG/RE PNPs) were synthesized by using simple ultrasonic irradiation method. The nanoparticles were characterized by using Fourier-transform infrared spectroscopy (FTIR) and scanning transmission electron microscopy (STEM). The viscosity behaviors of nanoparticles were studied in different conditions (pH, sonication time, and salt). The experimental results were calculated by Huggins, Kraemer, Tanglertpaibul-Rao, and Higiro models to understand the colloidal stability, the miscibility mechanism, and coefficients of nanoparticles. The results confirmed that the homogenous distribution of nanostructure was related to sonication time (30 min) and the presence of NaOH salt. With the addition of NaOH, the nanosystem based on ionotropic gelation technique was made more homogeneous. The results made us think that nanoparticles can be a good candidate for drug delivery systems in biomedical and pharmaceutical applications.

**Keywords:** ultrasonic-assisted, locust bean gum, rosin glycerol ester, polymeric nanoparticles

## 1. Introduction

Colloidal nanoparticles (CNPs) have attracted attention in industrial applications (food, pharmaceuticals, cosmetics, ink, rubber, and water treatment) due to their biological, mechanical, and thermal properties and stability in solution. Their superior properties depend on the high surface area, small size, and uniform morphologies [1–3]. CNPs are prepared to use different methods such as sol–gel [4], photochemical [5], electrochemical [6], laser ablation [7], ionizing irradiations [8], and ultrasonic irradiation [9].

The ultrasonic irradiation synthesis of different morphologies of nanomaterials consisted of metal/metal oxides, and polymeric materials have received considerable attention in the nanotechnology applications. The ultrasonic irradiation (20 kHz to 10 MHz) method has been employed in the preparation of the high purity, the uniform shape, and the nanosized distribution of nanomaterials.

This method causes the formation of the acoustic cavitations which consist of the bubbles [10]. The growth and collapse of bubbles are related to the transfer of energy at high pressures and temperatures due to the highly reactive free radicals such as hydrogen radicals (H•) and hydroxyl radicals (OH•). Bubbles generate three zones, such as a hot spot (5000°C, 500 atm), a gas–liquid interface (300°C, 50 atm), and a bulk solution (25°C, 1 atm) [11].

In recent research, different structures of nanoparticles such as $TiO_2$ [12], ZnO [13], starch [14], alumina/carbon core-shell [15], lipid-polymer hybrid [16], and biopolymeric [17, 18] nanoparticles have been synthesized with the ultrasonic irradiation method. Generally, biopolymeric nanoparticles have used in the field of foods encapsulation and drug delivery studies due to the biodegradability, biocompatibility, and low toxicity properties. Alginate [19], chitosan [20], carboxymethyl cellulose/gelatin [21], Senegal gum [22], guar gum [23], xanthan gum [24], *Senna tora* gum [25], and locust bean gum (LBG) [26] are natural biopolymers employed in industrial processes [24]. Locust bean gum is a neutral polysaccharide and has a mannose backbone with single side chain galactose units [25–27].

When the studies in the current literature are examined, it has been found that there are very few studies on LGB based on nanoparticles [28–30]. It was found that no studies were performed on the locust nanostructures containing rosin gum and derivatives. In this work, the ultrasonic irradiation method was used for the preparation of novel PEGylated locust bean gum (PEG-LBG)/rosin glycerol ester (RE) polymeric nanoparticles (PNPs) at room temperature. The present research work was aimed at the colloidal stability, the viscosity behaviour, and miscibility of binary polymer blends of PEG and LBG PNPs due to the intrinsic viscosity. The intrinsic viscosity of the polymer is a significant molecular characteristic, depending on the size of the polymer chain, molecular weight, and radius of rotation of the polymer in dilute solution. The voluminosity (VE), shape factor ($\upsilon$), the intrinsic viscosity $[\eta]$, and Krigbaum and Wall miscibility parameter ($\Delta b$) of polymeric nanoparticles were calculated from different models such as Huggins, Kraemer, Tanglertpaibul-Rao, and Higiro [17]. The values of intrinsic viscosities were used to determine the rheological behaviour of the PEG-LBG/RE PNPs at different conditions (pH, sonication time, and salt). The homogeneous distributions of PEG with LGB had an influence on the blends ratio of PEG/LBG (1:1, 1:2), sonication time (10–70 min.), temperature (25–35°C), and salts (NaOH, KOH, CTAB). With the addition of NaOH salt, PEG-LBG/RE PNPs based on ionotropic gelation technique were made into a more homogeneous solution. The PEG-LBG/RE PNPs were characterized to examine surface morphologies using a Fourier-transform infrared spectroscopy (FTIR) and scanning transmission electron microscopy (STEM). The aim of this study was to provide an investigation of rosin ester-based nanoparticle distributions in LGB and understand the role of polymer–particle interactions with respect to nanoparticle concentration as well to use the candidate nanocarrier for biomedical applications.

## 2. Materials and methods

### 2.1 Materials

Locust bean gum from *Ceratonia siliqua* seeds (M.W. of approx. 310 kDa) was purchased from Sigma Aldrich. Polyethylene glycol (PEG 400) was obtained from Fluka (Switzerland). Ethyl acetate (anhydrous, 99.8%) was purchased from Sigma Aldrich. Dimethyl sulfoxide (DMSO), potassium hydroxide (KOH), sodium hydroxide (NaOH), and cetyltrimethylammonium bromide (CTAB) were purchased from Merck. Rosin glycerol ester was purchased from Pina Kimya (CAS: 8050-26-8, EC: 232–479-9, Turkey). All other reagents and chemicals were of analytical grade.

### 2.2 Preparation of PEG-LBG/RE polymeric nanoparticles

PEG-LBG/RE PNPs were synthesized using the ultrasonic irradiation method (Ultrasonics Vibra-Cell, probe type, amplitude %30, a frequency of 20 kHz) with different ratios of blends (PEG-LBG: 1:1, 1:2). In the procedure, two phases were prepared such as the dispersion phase and the continuous phase.

*The continuous phase*: 125 mg LBG was dissolved in 50 ml of distilled water (60°C for 20 min) and then added to 125 mg of PEG400 polymer solution at room temperature.

*The dispersion phase*: 0.01 g RE was dissolved in 0.5 ml DMSO and then 7 ml ethyl acetate was added to the solution.

7.5 ml of continuous phase and the dispersed phase was sonicated at room temperature. 42.5 ml of continuous phase was then added slowly to the blends, and the sonication procedure was continued for 30 minutes. The final solution was evaporated at room temperature for 14 hours until ethyl acetate completely evaporated in the solution. Polymer blends were also performed for different composition ratios (PEG-LBG) such as 1:1 and 1:2.

### 2.3 Characterization parts

The dynamics viscosities of LBG, PEG-LBG, and PEG-LBG/RE were determined by a programmable AND viscometer (SV-10, Sine-wave Vibro Viscometer, A $\delta$ D Company). PEG-LBG/RE PNPs were scanned in the dark field area with the wet STEM detector by using FEI QUANTA S50 (A copper grid, Ted Pella, support films, carbon type A, 300 meshes was utilized). STEM holder was cooled to 2°C and the pressure was set between 700 and 1300 Pa. Samples were ground with KBr powder and analyzed from 4000 to 600 $cm^{-1}$ with a resolution of 4 $cm^{-1}$ using 8 scans by using a PerkinElmer FTIR emission spectrometer.

### 2.4 Calculations of the multi-concentration regression models

The changes in viscosity values of LBG, PEG-LBG, and PEG-LBG/RE PNPs were investigated in a dilute solution (50 mL) at different ratios of polymer blends (PEG-LBG: 1:1 and 1:2), temperatures (25 and 35°C), and sonication times (10–70 min) in

| | | Formula | Ref: |
|---|---|---|---|
| Specific viscosity | $\eta_{sp} = \frac{t}{t_0} - 1$ | (1) | [31] |
| Intrinsic viscosity | $[\eta] = \lim_{C \to 0} \left(\frac{\eta_{sp}}{C}\right)$ | (2) | [31] |
| | Multi-concentration regression models: | | |
| Huggins | $\eta_{sp}/C = [\eta] + k_1[\eta]^2 C$ ($k_1$, Huggins constant) | (3) | [32] |
| Kraemer | $In\ \eta_{rel}/C = [\eta] + k_2[\eta]^2 C$ ($k_2$, Kraemer constant) | (4) | [33] |
| Tanglertpaibul-Rao | $\eta_{rel} = 1 + [\eta]C$ | (5) | [34] |
| Higiro | $\eta_{rel} = e^{[\eta]C}$ | (6) | [28] |

**Table 1.**
*The equations of the intrinsic viscosity, the specific viscosity, and the multi-concentration regression models.*

the presence of NaOH, KOH, and CTAB salts. The specific viscosities ($\eta_{sp}$), the intrinsic viscosities ([η]), and the multi-concentration regression models of PEG-LBG/RE PNPs were calculated by using an AND viscometer (WinCT-Viscosity software) in 50 ml solution at constant temperature [31–36] (**Table 1**).

In this study, the voluminosity (VE), shape factor (υ), and Krigbaum and Wall parameter ($\Delta b$) were calculated using the following Eqs. 7–10, respectively. The polymer blends are miscible if $\Delta b \geq 0$ and immiscible when $\Delta b < 0$. ($b_{12}^{*}$, the experimental interaction parameter; $b_{12}$, the theoretical interaction parameter):

$$\gamma = \frac{\eta_{rel}^{0.5} - 1}{C\left(1.35\eta_{rel}^{0.5} - 0.1\right)} \tag{7}$$

$$[\eta] = \upsilon V_E \tag{8}$$

$$b_{12}^{*} = \sqrt{b_{11}b_{22}} \tag{9}$$

$$\Delta b = b_{12} - b_{12}^{*} \tag{10}$$

## 3. Results and discussions

### 3.1 Colloidal stability and viscosity analysis

#### *3.1.1 The multi-concentration regression models and salt factor*

The intrinsic viscosity of [η] of PEG, LBG, PEG-LBG (1:1), and PEG-LBG/RE 1:1 nanoparticles was calculated using the multi-concentration regression models (Huggins, Kraemer, Tanglertpaibul-Rao, and Higiro models) at room temperatures. The correlation coefficient ($R^2$), the intrinsic viscosity, and parameters of Huggins,

| | Huggins | | | Kraemer | | | Tanglertpaibul-Rao | | Higiro | |
|---|---|---|---|---|---|---|---|---|---|---|
| **pH** | **[η] (ml/g)** | **$k_1 \times 10^{-3}$** | **$R^2$** | **[η] (ml/g)** | **$k_2$** | **$R^2$** | **[η] (ml/g)** | **$R^2$** | **[η] (ml/g)** | **$R^2$** |
| A | 4.70 | 0.213 | 0.99 | 6.73 | 1.129 | 0.89 | 9.11 | 0.96 | 10.87 | 0.98 |
| B | 5.18 | 0.193 | 0.99 | 56.75 | −0.075 | 0.87 | 41.32 | 0.98 | 12.68 | 0.99 |
| C | 2.25 | 0.445 | 0.96 | 71.95 | −0.067 | 0.86 | 41.57 | 1.00 | 12.65 | 0.99 |
| D | 0.67 | 1.493 | 0.99 | 55.78 | −0.073 | 0.87 | 43.94 | 1.00 | 10.97 | 0.99 |

*Samples: (A) PEG, (B) LBG, (C) PEG-LBG/ (1:1), (D) PEG-LBG/RE (1:2), and (E) PEG-LBG/RE (1:1).*

**Table 2.**
*The intrinsic viscosity (ml/g) values of PEG-LBG blends and PEG-LBG/RE nanoparticles at room temperature for different concentrations.*

| | **$V_E$ (ml/g)** | **$\upsilon$** | | **Δb $(mL/g)^2$** | **Miscibility** |
|---|---|---|---|---|---|
| PEG-LBG (1:1) | 38 | 2.5> | spherical | 1.59 | Miscible |
| **PEG-LBG/RE PNPs (1:2)** | **42** | — | | −0.64 | İmmiscible |
| PEG-LBG/RE PNPs (1:1) | 35 | 2.5 > | spherical | 1.56 | Miscible |

**Table 3.**
*Voluminosity and shape factor of LBG, PEG-LBG, and PEG-LBG/RE PNPs.*

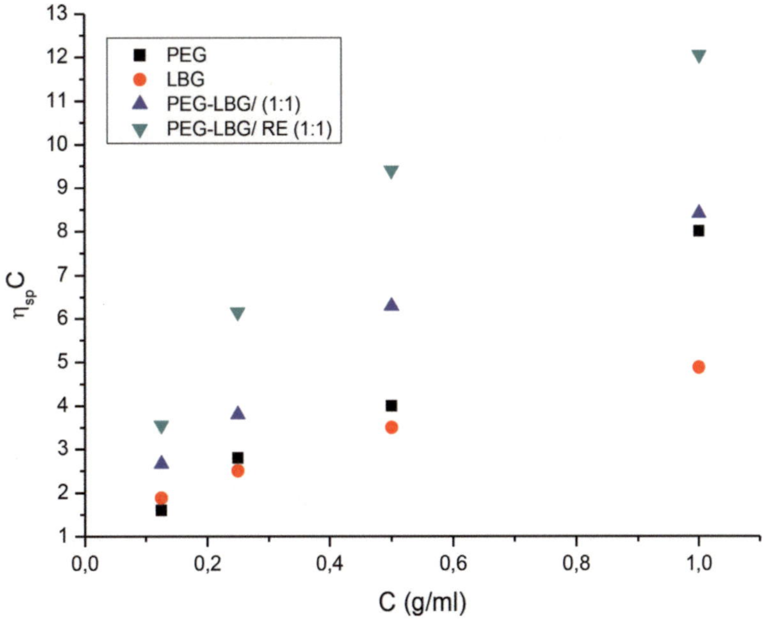


**Figure 1.**
*The Huggins plots of PEG, LBG, PEG-LBG (1:1), and PEG-LBG/RE PNPs.*

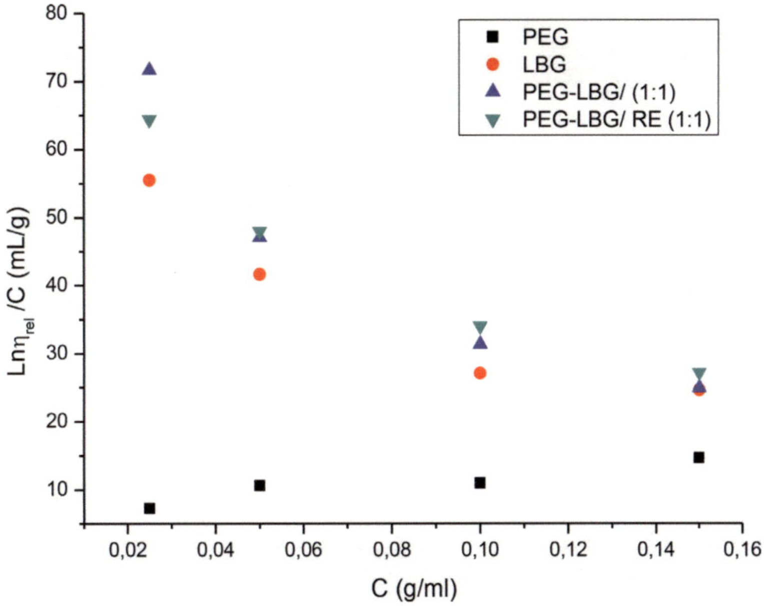


**Figure 2.**
*The Kraemer plots of PEG, LBG, PEG-LBG (1:1), and PEG-LBG/RE PNPs.*

Kraemer, Tanglertpaibul-Rao, and Higiro models were given comparatively in **Table 2** (**Figures 1–4**). In this study, we focused on the effect of nanoparticles on the morphology of immiscible polymer blends. We found that PEG-LBG/RE PNPs (1:2) were immiscible due to the mixing ratio of PEG-LBG (**Table 3**).

The Huggins, Kraemer, Tanglertpaibul-Rao, and Higiro plots of the intrinsic viscosities were calculated at different blend ratios, and the results showed the critical role on relation between the intrinsic viscosities and the blend ratios.

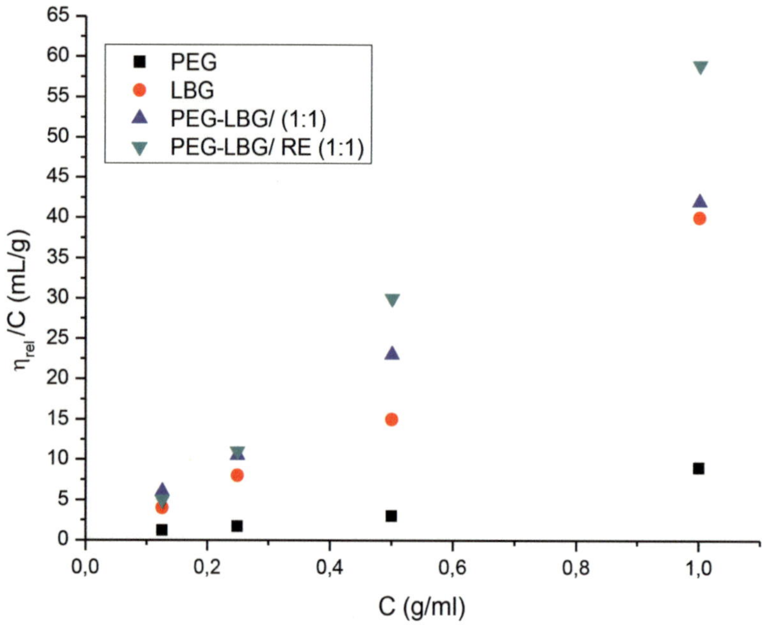


**Figure 3.**
*The Tanglertpaibul-Rao's plots of PEG, LBG, PEG-LBG (1:1), and PEG-LBG/RE PNPs.*

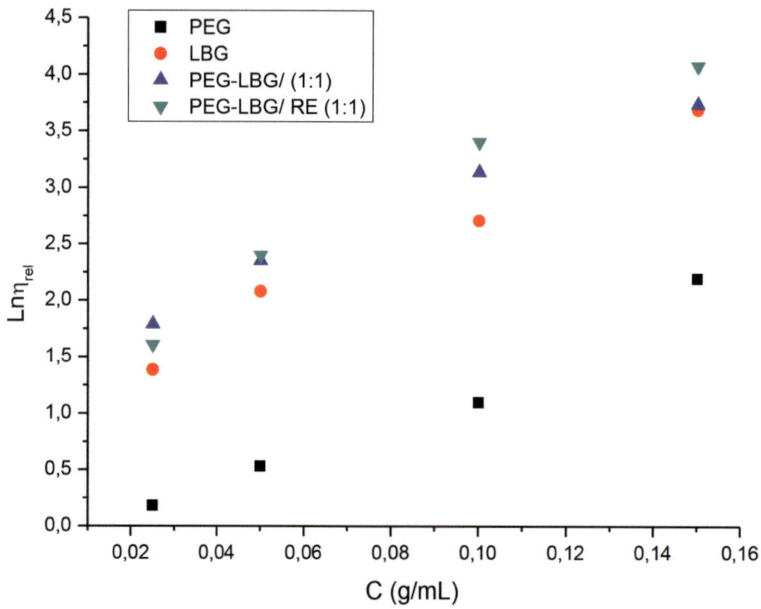


**Figure 4.**
*The Higiro plots of PEG, LBG, PEG-LBG (1:1), and PEG-LBG/RE PNPs.*

The Tanglertpaibul-Rao model and Huggins model ($R^2$ = 0.96–1.00) were the best models to understand the intrinsic viscosity of PEG, LBG, PEG-LBG, and PEG-LBG/RE PNPs. Behrouzian et al. [32] reported that the Tanglertpaibul and Rao model was the best model for the intrinsic viscosity determination of cress seed gum

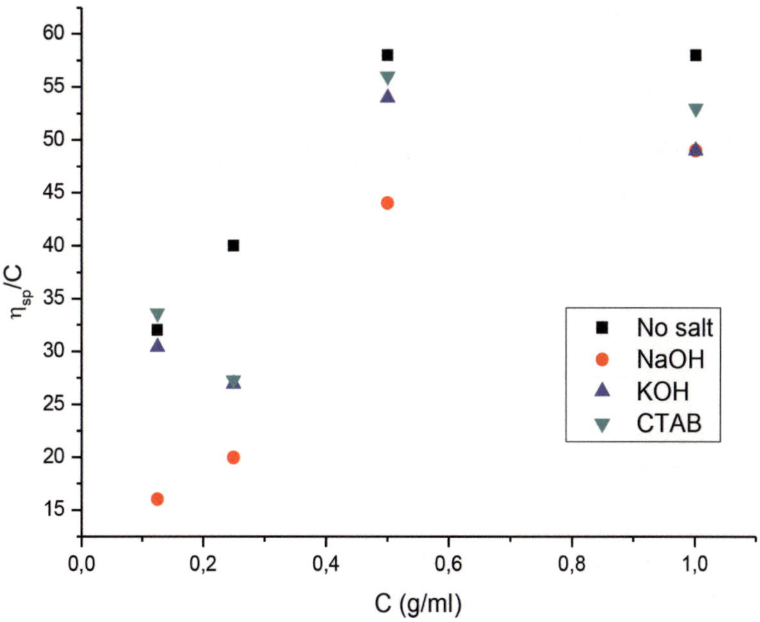


**Figure 5.**
*Plots of the intrinsic viscosity versus C of PEG-LBG/RE PNPs in the presence of salts (KOH, NaOH, and CTAB).*

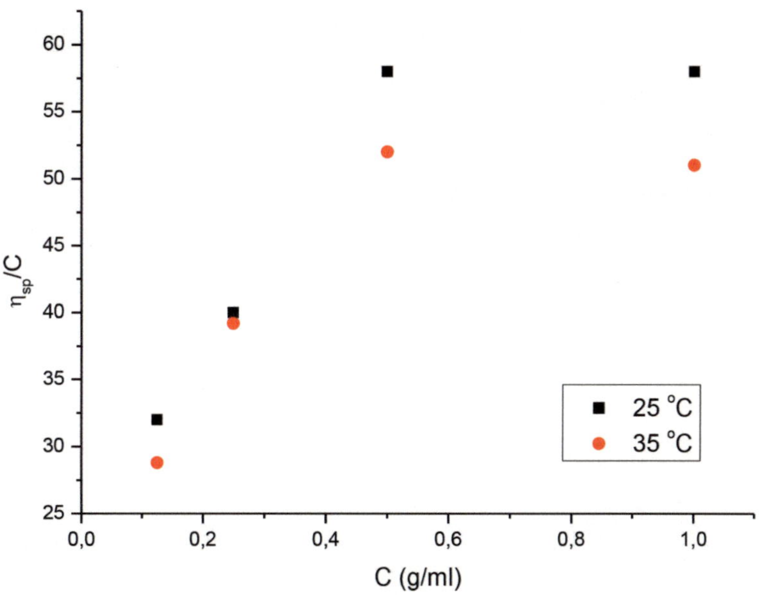


**Figure 6.**
*Plots of [η] of PEG-LBG/RE PNPs at different temperatures (25 and 35°C).*

solutions. Razavi et al. [37] reported that the best model was Tanglertpaibul and Rao model for wild sage seed gum. In this study, the intrinsic viscosity of PEG-LBG/RE PNPs in the presence of different salts (NaOH, KOH, and CTAB) was investigated (Csalt, 0.1 M; Vsalt, 2 mL; Vsolution; 50 mL) at 25°C. The effect of NaOH, KOH, and CTAB salts on the values of intrinsic viscosity of PEG-LBG/RE PNPs (1:1) was presented in **Figure 5**.

The pH values of the solutions (LBG, PEG-LBG, and PEG-LBG/RE PNPs) at initial pH in KOH, NaOH, and CTAB salt additions were determined: $pH_{initial}$, 5.7; $pH_{initial}$, 5.55; and $pH_{initial}$, 5.32, respectively. In the presence of salt, the values of the intrinsic viscosity for the mixture were observed to change in two different salts such as KOH ($pH_{final:}$ 5.93) and NaOH ($pH_{final}$: 5.72). The [η] values for PEG-LBG/RE PNPs (1:1) did not exhibit distinctive changes in the presence of CTAB ($pH_{final}$: 3.87). Jiang et al. [38] reported that the interactions between blends were dependent on the ionic strength at low salt concentration which was related to the increase of salt concentration. Consequently the addition of NaOH and KOH showed the electrostatic repulsion between charges along the backbone of the polymer blends.

### *3.1.2 Temperature and sonication time factor*

The intrinsic viscosity decreased when the temperature increased, and the relation of the experimental results of PEG-LBG/RE PNPs with the temperature was shown in **Figure 6**.

However, when PEG-LBG/RE PNPs were sonicated, the intrinsic viscosity decreased for 30 minutes but remained constant after a period of time. These results had proven that the sonication time changed the value of viscosity and was effective on the blends (30% amp., 25°C) (**Figure** 7). The viscosity of Cu-ethylene glycol (EG) nanofluids was proven to decrease with the sonication time [39]. In this study, we found a similar situation, and demonstrated that sonication time changes the viscosity, which has a role on the formation of nanoparticles.

### *3.1.3 The voluminosity, shape factor, and miscibility parameter*

In this study, we investigated the relationship between the intrinsic viscosity and the surface morphology, particle size, and shape. The shape factor was calculated using the approach given as follows: (a) $n < 2.5$ indicates spherical shape, and (b) $n > 2.5$ indicates ellipsoidal particles [40].

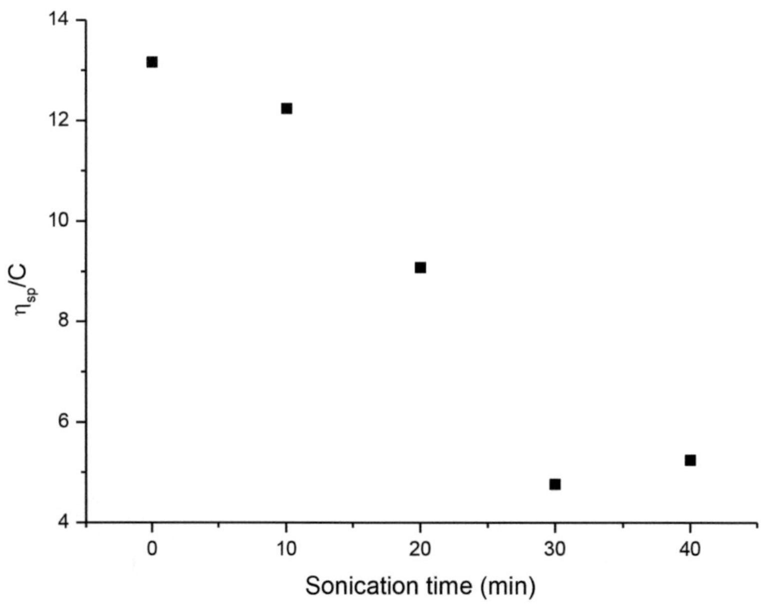


**Figure 7.**
*Plots of [η] of PEG-LBG/RE PNPs at different sonication times (30% amp., 25°C).*

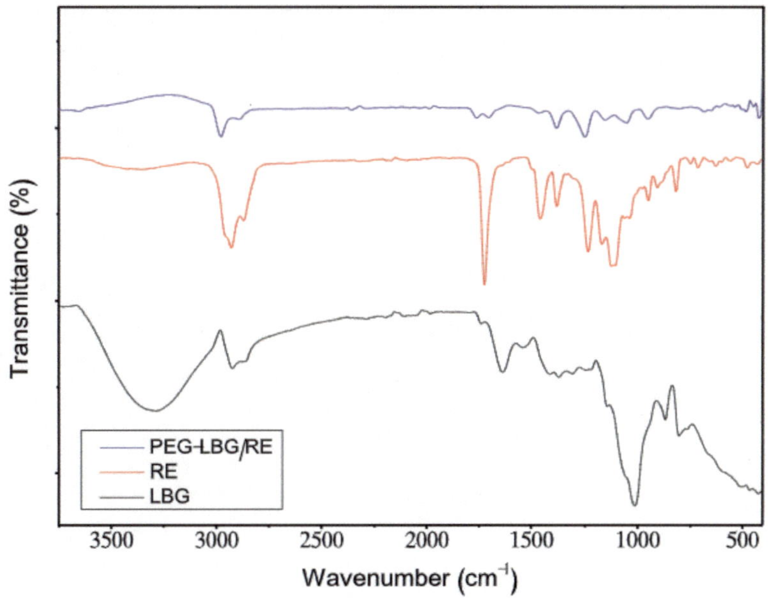


**Figure 8.**
*The FTIR spectrum of pure LBG, pure RE, and PEG-LBG/RE PNPs.*

In this study, we predicted the size and shape factor of PEG-LBG (1:1), PEG-LBG/RE PNPs (1:1), and PEG-LBG/RE PNPs (1:2) using the values of the intrinsic viscosity, associated with the shape factor, which were used to determine the change in the structure configuration. We calculated the shape and the Krigbaum and Wall (Δb) parameters of PEG-LBG/RE PNPs (1:1) using the intrinsic viscosity to determine the changes in the blends. We found that PEG-LBG/RE PNPs (1:1) had a spherical-like configuration, and the amounts of PEG had a role on the miscibility due to the interactions between the functional groups in the blends.

### 3.2 FTIR analysis

The FTIR spectra of pure LBG, pure RE, and PEG-LBG/RE PNPs were shown in **Figure 8**.

The FTIR spectrum of pure LBG showed a broad absorption peak at 3250 $cm^{-1}$ (stretching of -OH group), 2952 $cm^{-1}$ (stretching of –CH), 1748 $cm^{-1}$ (stretching of C=O), and 1000–1100 $cm^{-1}$ (stretching of C-O-H). Upadhyay et al. [41] and Chakravorty et al. [42] found the FTIR spectrum data similar. The FTIR spectrum of pure RE showed a peak at 3330 $cm^{-1}$ (stretching of -OH group), 1730 $cm^{-1}$ (stretching of C=O), and 1120 $cm^{-1}$ (stretching of C-O-H). As we have seen from the FTIR results, we have demonstrated that the apparent OH peak of LBG disappeared and that the rosin glycerol ester is coated with surrounding PEGylated LBG.

### 3.3 STEM analysis

According to the STEM image of PEG-LBG/RE PNPs (160.000x and 300.000x), we can see that the interior structure of the polymeric nanoparticle is LBG with the size lower than 50 nm. We are able to tell that these particles are small agglomerates of it (**Figure 9**).

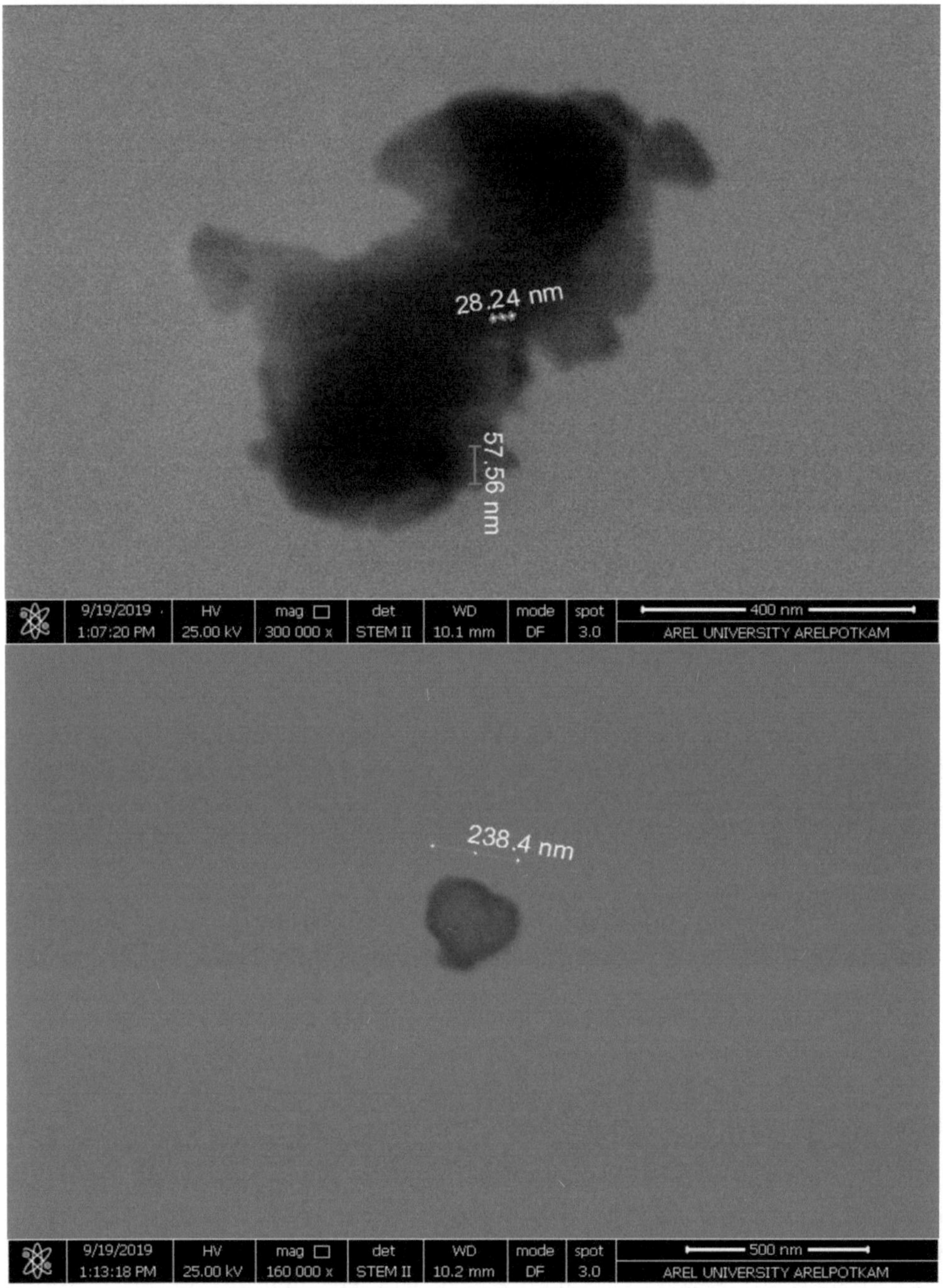


**Figure 9.**
*STEM image of PEG-LBG/RE PNPs (160.000x and 300.000x).*

## 4. Conclusions

We prepared the novel PEG-LBG/RE PNPs with an average particle size of 100 nm using the ultrasonic irradiation. We dispersed the amphiphilic RE coated with PEG-LBG blends in nanosize and spherical structure. We focused on the miscibility of the blends, and shapes of the polymeric nanoparticles were calculated using the values of the intrinsic viscosity in different conditions. We estimate that

PEG-LBG/RE PNPs can be used to increase the therapeutic efficacy and biocompatibility of the nanodrug in pharmaceutical and biomedical studies.

## Acknowledgements

The authors acknowledge the STEM and FTIR analysis support from Arel POTKAM (Istanbul, Turkey), Zeynep Akça, Demet SEZGİN MANSUROGLU, and Deniz ISMIK.

## Author details

Selcan Karakus[1*], Merve Ilgar[1], Ezgi Tan[1], Yeşim Müge Sahin[2,3], Nevin Tasaltin[4] and Ayben Kilislioglu[1]

1 Department of Chemistry, Faculty of Engineering, Istanbul University-Cerrahpasa, Istanbul, Turkey

2 ArelPOTKAM, Polymer Technologies and Composite Application and Research Center, Istanbul Arel University, Istanbul, Turkey

3 Department of Biomedical Engineering, Faculty of Engineering and Architecture, Istanbul Arel University, Istanbul, Turkey

4 Department of Electrical-Electronics Engineering, Maltepe University, Istanbul, Turkey

*Address all correspondence to: selcan@istanbul.edu.tr

## References

[1] Montasser I, Fessi H, Coleman AW. Atomic force microscopy imaging of novel type of polymeric colloidal nanostructures. European Journal of Pharmaceutics and Biopharmaceutics. 2002;**54**(3):281-284

[2] Bourgeat-Lami E. Organic–inorganic nanostructured colloids. Journal of Nanoscience and Nanotechnology. 2002;**2**(1):1-24

[3] Petry R, Saboia VM, Franqui LS, Holanda CA, Garcia TR, de Farias G, et al. On the formation of protein corona on colloidal nanoparticles stabilized by depletant polymers. Materials Science and Engineering: C.18. 2019;**105**:1-12

[4] Behnajady MA, Eskandarloo H, Modirshahla N, Shokri M. Sol-gel low temperature synthesis of stable anatase type $TiO_2$ nanoparticles under different conditions and its photocatalytic activity. Photochemistry and Photobiology. 2011;**87**(5):1002-1008

[5] Henglein A. Colloidal silver nanoparticles: Photochemical preparation and interaction with $O_2$, $CC_{14}$, and some metal ions. Chemistry of Materials. 1998;**10**(1):444-450

[6] Cabrera L, Gutierrez S, Menendez N, Morales MP, Herrasti P. Magnetite nanoparticles: Electrochemical synthesis and characterization. Electrochimica Acta. 2008;**53**(8):3436-3441

[7] Im HJ, Jung EC. Colloidal nanoparticles produced from Cu metal in water by laser ablation and their agglomeration. Radiation Physics and Chemistry. 2016;**118**:6-10

[8] Gasaymeh SS, Radiman S, Heng LY, Saion E, Saeed GM. Synthesis and characterization of silver/polyvinilpirrolidone (Ag/PVP) nanoparticles using gamma irradiation techniques. The African Review of Physics. 2010;**4**:31-41

[9] Tan E, Karakus S, Soylu GSP, Birer Ö, Zengin Y, Kilislioglu A. Formation and distribution of ZnO nanoparticles and its effect on E. coli in the presence of sepiolite and silica within the chitosan matrix via sonochemistry. Ultrasonics Sonochemistry. 2017;**38**:720-725

[10] Gong C, Hart DP. Ultrasound induced cavitation and sonochemical yields. The Journal of the Acoustical Society of America. 1998;**104**(5):2675-2682

[11] Cui D, Mebel AM, Arroyo-Mora LE, Holness H, Furton KG, O'Shea K. Kinetic, product, and computational studies of the ultrasonic induced degradation of 4-methylcyclohexanemethanol (MCHM). Water Research. 2017;**126**:164-171

[12] Masoudian N, Rajabi M, Ghaedi M. Titanium oxide nanoparticles loaded onto activated carbon prepared from bio-waste watermelon rind for the efficient ultrasonic-assisted adsorption of Congo red and phenol red dyes from wastewaters. Polyhedron. 2019;**173**:1-9

[13] Karakuş S. Preparation and rheological characterization of Chitosan-Gelatine@ ZnO-Si nanoparticles. International Journal of Biological Macromolecules. 2019;**137**:821-828

[14] Boufi S, Haaj SB, Magnin A, Pignon F, Impéror-Clerc M, Mortha G. Ultrasonic assisted production of starch nanoparticles: Structural characterization and mechanism of disintegration. Ultrasonics Sonochemistry. 2018;**41**:327-336

[15] Sabaghi V, Davar F, Taherian MH. Ultrasonic-assisted preparation of AlON from alumina/carbon core-shell nanoparticle. Ceramics International. 2019;**45**(3):3350-3358

[16] Dave V, Tak K, Sohgaura A, Gupta A, Sadhu V, Reddy KR. Lipid-polymer hybrid nanoparticles: Synthesis strategies and biomedical applications. Journal of Microbiological Methods. 2019;**160**:130-142

[17] Karakus S, Ilgar M, Kahyaoglu IM, Kilislioglu A. Influence of ultrasound irradiation on the intrinsic viscosity of guar gum–PEG/rosin glycerol ester nanoparticles. International Journal of Biological Macromolecules. 2019;**141**: 1118-1127

[18] Barak S, Mudgil D. Locust bean gum: Processing, properties and food applications—A review. International Journal of Biological Macromolecules. 2014;**66**:74-80

[19] Jayapal JJ, Dhanaraj S. Exemestane loaded alginate nanoparticles for cancer treatment: Formulation and in vitro evaluation. International Journal of Biological Macromolecules. 2017;**105**: 416-421

[20] Yu S, Xu X, Feng J, Liu M, Hu K. Chitosan and chitosan coating nanoparticles for the treatment of brain disease. International Journal of Pharmaceutics. 2019;**560**:282-293

[21] Sethi S, Kaith BS, Kumar V. Fabrication and characterization of microwave assisted carboxymethyl cellulose-gelatin silver nanoparticles imbibed hydrogel: Its evaluation as dye degradation. Reactive and Functional Polymers. 2019;**142**:134-146

[22] Şişmanoğlu T, Karakuş S, Birer Ö, Soylu GSP, Kolan A, Tan E, et al. Preparation and characterization of antibacterial Senegalia (Acacia) Senegal/iron–silica bio-nanocomposites. Applied Surface Science. 2015;**354**: 250-255

[23] Patra AS, Ghorai S, Ghosh S, Mandal B, Pal S. Selective removal of toxic anionic dyes using a novel nanocomposite derived from cationically modified guar gum and silica nanoparticles. Journal of Hazardous Materials. 2016;**301**:127-136

[24] Pooja D, Panyaram S, Kulhari H, Rachamalla SS, Sistla R. Xanthan gum stabilized gold nanoparticles: Characterization, biocompatibility, stability and cytotoxicity. Carbohydrate Polymers. 2014;**110**:1-9

[25] Braz L, Grenha A, Ferreira D, da Costa AMR, Gamazo C, Sarmento B. Chitosan/sulfated locust bean gum nanoparticles: In vitro and in vivo evaluation towards an application in oral immunization. International Journal of Biological Macromolecules. 2017;**96**:786-797

[26] Pawar HA, Lalitha KG, Ruckmani K. Alginate beads of captopril using galactomannan containing Senna tora gum, guar gum and locust bean gum. International Journal of Biological Macromolecules. 2015;**76**:119-131

[27] Perestrelo AR, Grenha A, da Costa AMR, Belo JA. Locust bean gum as an alternative polymeric coating for embryonic stem cell culture. Materials Science and Engineering: C. 2014;**40**: 336-344

[28] Higiro J, Herald TJ, Alavi S, Bean S. Rheological study of xanthan and locust bean gum interaction in dilute solution: Effect of salt. Food Research International. 2007;**40**(4):435-447

[29] Cordeiro T, Paninho AB, Bernardo M, Matos I, Pereira CV, Serra AT, et al. Biocompatible locust bean gum as mesoporous carriers for naproxen delivery. Materials Chemistry and Physics. 2020;**239**:121973

[30] Braz L, Grenha A, Corvo MC, Lourenco JP, Ferreira D, Sarmento B, et al. Synthesis and characterization of locust bean gum derivatives and their

application in the production of nanoparticles. Carbohydrate Polymers. 2018;**181**:974-985

[31] Soumya RS, Sherin S, Raghu KG, Abraham A. Allicin functionalized locust bean gum nanoparticles for improved therapeutic efficacy: An in silico, in vitro and in vivo approach. International Journal of Biological Macromolecules. 2018;**109**:740-747

[32] Behrouzian F, Razavi SM, Karazhiyan H. Intrinsic viscosity of cress (*Lepidium sativum*) seed gum: Effect of salts and sugars. Food Hydrocolloids. 2014;**35**:100-105

[33] Huggins ML. The viscosity of dilute solutions of long-chain molecules. IV. Dependence on concentration. Journal of the American Chemical Society. 1942; **64**(11):2716-2718

[34] Kraemer EO. Molecular weights of cellulose and cellulose derivatives. Industrial & Engineering Chemistry. 1938;**30**(10):1200-1203

[35] Tanglertpaibul T, Rao MA. Intrinsic viscosity of tomato serum as affected by methods of determination and methods of processing concentrates. Journal of Food Science. 1987;**52**(6):1642-1645

[36] Chen HH, Kang HY, Chen SD. The effects of ingredients and water content on the rheological properties of batters and physical properties of crusts in fried foods. Journal of Food Engineering. 2008;**88**(1):45-54

[37] Razavi SM, Moghaddam TM, Emadzadeh B, Salehi F. Dilute solution properties of wild sage (*Salvia macrosiphon*) seed gum. Food Hydrocolloids. 2012;**29**(1):205-210

[38] Jiang WH, Han SJ. The interactions of chitosan–poly (ethylene glycol) in the presence of added salt in water: Viscosity effect. European Polymer Journal. 1999;**35**(11):2079-2085

[39] Li F, Li L, Zhong G, Zhai Y, Li Z. Effects of ultrasonic time, size of aggregates and temperature on the stability and viscosity of Cu-ethylene glycol (EG) nanofluids. International Journal of Heat and Mass Transfer. 2019;**129**:278-286

[40] Curvale R, Masuelli M, Padilla AP. Intrinsic viscosity of bovine serum albumin conformers. International Journal of Biological Macromolecules. 2008;**42**(2):133-137

[41] Upadhyay M, Adena SKR, Vardhan H, Yadav SK, Mishra B. Locust bean gum and sodium alginate based interpenetrating polymeric network microbeads encapsulating Capecitabine: Improved pharmacokinetics, cytotoxicity &in vivo antitumor activity. Materials Science and Engineering: C. 2019;**104**:109958

[42] Chakravorty A, Barman G, Mukherjee S, Sa B. Effect of carboxymethylation on rheological and drug release characteristics of locust bean gum matrix tablets. Carbohydrate Polymers. 2016;**144**:50-58

Chapter 2

# Magnetic and Quantum Dot Nanoparticles for Drug Delivery and Diagnostic Systems

*Erandi Munasinghe, Maheshi Aththapaththu and Lakmal Jayarathne*

## Abstract

Nanoparticles are being used tremendously in biomedical sciences due to their promising chemical and physical properties. Magnetic nanoparticles and quantum dot nanocrystals are two of the main nanoparticle types used in the biomedical industry. The surface of these nanoparticles is further modified in order to obtain biocompatibility and surface functionalization. Magnetic properties, fluorescence, nanometer size, and availability of sites to modify its surface for bioconjugation provide greater potential to use these nanoparticles in targeted drug delivery technique and diagnostics. As a result, these nanoparticles create massive developments in the industrial operations. In this chapter, an overview of the nanoparticles used in drug delivery and diagnostic systems will be discussed. In addition, advantages in encapsulation of magnetic and quantum dot nanoparticles for bioconjugation and different methods of drug delivery will be addressed.

**Keywords:** drug delivery, quantum dots, magnetic nanoparticles

## 1. Introduction

Among many synthetic compounds the general public comes across with, in day-to-day life, nanoparticles are considered highly advantageous in various applications. Nanoparticles in diagnostics and as drug delivery vehicles are coming under the aforementioned beneficial applications in the field of biomedical science. Various types of nanoparticles, for instance, gold nanoparticles [1] and iron oxide nanoparticles [2], are being used in biomedical operations. Due to its magnetic properties and nanometer size, magnetic nanoparticles such as magnetite ($Fe_3O_4$) [3] and maghemite ($\gamma$-$Fe_2O_3$) [4, 5] are considered highly beneficial for diagnostics and in drug delivery systems. On the other hand, inorganic nanoscale particles with semiconductor properties are becoming very popular in such applications. These semiconductor nanoparticles, called quantum dot nanoparticles, are equipped with extremely favorable characteristics such as high fluorescence and photoluminescence. These nanoparticles have been tested to be used in diagnostics [6], and trials were carried out at laboratory scale as therapeutics, that is, for drug delivery [7]. At the same time, quantum dots are found to be more beneficial over regular chemotherapy, radiation, and ionizing radiation imaging [8] which are used in cancer diagnosis and treatment.

 IntechOpen

## 2. Nanoparticles used in drug delivery and diagnostic systems

### 2.1 Magnetic nanoparticles

Magnetic nanoparticles are used widely in a variety of industrial applications in environmental remediation [9], data storage [10], electronic device development [11], and pharmaceutical industry [12, 13]. Its magnetic properties give a greater potential in delivering the drugs at desired sites. The nanoscale size of the particles gives the ability to permeate through membranes without the interference of biological barriers. Therefore, the so-called properties make magnetic nanoparticles an ineluctable component in the development of drug delivery systems.

#### *2.1.1 Properties of magnetic nanoparticles*

Several types of magnetic nanoparticles such as iron, nickel, and cobalt based are available for industrial applications [14]. Due to the greater potential in surface modification and higher magnetic properties, iron oxide nanoparticles are considered as the best magnetic candidate in the development of drug delivery systems. These single-domain iron oxide magnetic nanoparticles are present in three different phases, as magnetite, maghemite, and hematite ($\alpha$-$Fe_2O_3$) [15]. These nanoparticles generally demonstrate super-paramagnetic properties at ambient conditions even though their physical and chemical properties largely depend on the synthesis procedure and particle size [16]. According to the motions and interactions of the electrons available in the material, magnetism is divided in to five main classes as diamagnetism, paramagnetism, ferrimagnetism, ferromagnetism, and antiferromagnetism [17, 18]. Iron oxide nanoparticles fall under ferromagnetic and ferromagnetic classes due to their strong collective magnetic interaction [18].

To be used in a biological environment, there are several concerns that the magnetic nanoparticles should conquer. Colloidal and chemical stability of these particles is the main consideration. The stability of magnetic nanoparticles is extremely affected by intrinsic structural properties such as size, morphology, and pH of the particles [19].

#### *2.1.2 Synthesis of magnetic nanoparticles*

Synthesis of iron oxide nanoparticles can be conducted in different procedures using physical, chemical, or biological methods [18]. Chemical methods such as coprecipitation, hydrothermal reactions, thermal decomposition, microemulsion, sol-gel reactions, aerosol/vapor phase method, and electrochemical method are the principal preparation procedures. These procedures have the ability to control particle size, surface chemistry, and composition. Most simple, efficient, and cost-effective methods among these procedures are coprecipitation and thermal decomposition, which are also used widely due to the same reasons. In coprecipitation, metal oxide particles are synthesized using a solution of the metal salt. In the synthesis of iron oxide nanoparticles, aqueous $Fe^{3+}$ and $Fe^{2+}$ are coprecipitated by addition of a base, preferably, sodium hydroxide or ammonium [18].

#### *2.1.3 Biomedical applications*

As a result of its nanometer size, as small as 3 nm [20], magnetic nanoparticles can reach the biological entities according to the interest. Cells with 10–100 μm size, proteins as large as 5–50 nm or even genes which can be 2 nm wide and 10–100 nm long, or viruses with size ranging from 20 to 450 nm can be targeted using these magnetic nanoparticles [21]. The property of magnetism, where these nanoparticles can be manipulated by an external magnetic field, enhances its utility by providing the ability to get these nanoparticles to where they are required. Magnetic nanoparticles are used in various applications in the aspects of biomedicine and biology. Magnetic separation has been of greater advantage in biological research, where magnetic nanoparticles are labeled to desired biological substances. These have proven superior sensitivity in cell sorting especially in immuno-magnetic selection of rare tumor cells in blood [22]. Moreover, these magnetic nanoparticles are used in a vast number of biological operations such as targeted drug delivery [23], hyperthermia [24], magnetic resonance imaging (MRI) [25], rapid diagnostics [26], tissue engineering [27], magnetic particle imaging (MPI) [28], etc.

## 2.2 Quantum dot nanoparticles

Quantum dot nanocrystals are semiconductor nanomaterials with intrinsic chemical and physical properties. These have unique semiconductor energy levels that can be adopted by simply changing size, shape, and charge potential [29]. In quantum dot nanoparticles, excitons are confined in all three dimensions. Quantum confinement is a property of semiconductors where the diameter of the nanoparticle approaches that of the Bohr exciton radius. These nanoparticles have particular optical and electronic properties such as size-tunable absorption bands and emission colors due to the quantum confinement effect [30]. Quantum dot particles are artificially synthesized from II to IV and III to V elements such as Cd, Te, Se, Zn, etc. [31]. These are nanoscale structures typically with a diameter of 2–10 nm, which make them a more reliable and influential candidate in most of the industrial applications. Due to its small diameter, the surface atom to core atom ratio is high [32]. When the surface atom to core atom ratio increases, the properties of surface atoms dominate the properties of the whole particle. The semiconductor lattice of quantum dots is terminating on the surface, and therefore, the surface atoms show a different chemical behavior than the core atoms [33]. This ultimately makes the quantum dots more beneficial in industrial and biomedical operations.

### *2.2.1 Properties of quantum dot nanoparticles*

These nanocrystals display fluorescence and produce distinctive colors which can be determined by the nanocrystal particle size. Fluorescence is a form of luminescence, where a substance absorbs light or other electromagnetic radiation and emits light of a longer wavelength than the absorbed light [34]. In general, luminescence is defined as the emission of photons from the excited electronic state. In contrast, when the atoms of the material absorb energy, these atoms are in the excited state. These excited atoms release absorbed energy as photons, which ultimately discharge light [35]. These quantum dot nanoparticles exhibit extraordinary photoluminescence with increased brightness and stability [36, 37].

As presented in **Figure 1**, there are several types of quantum dots as core type [38], core-shell type [39], and alloyed type (bimetallic) [40], which are classified based on their composition and structure. Core-type quantum dots contain single component inorganic core and can be chalcogenides of metals such as PbS, CdTe, CdSe, etc. [38]. These can be further modified with another layer around the core using many substances, according to the application's requirement. Typically, in biomedical applications, these core structures are stabilized with an organic layer around the core in order to obtain a hydrophobic or hydrophilic surface. The electroluminescent and photoluminescent properties of these core-type quantum dots can be refined by basically altering the crystal size [12].

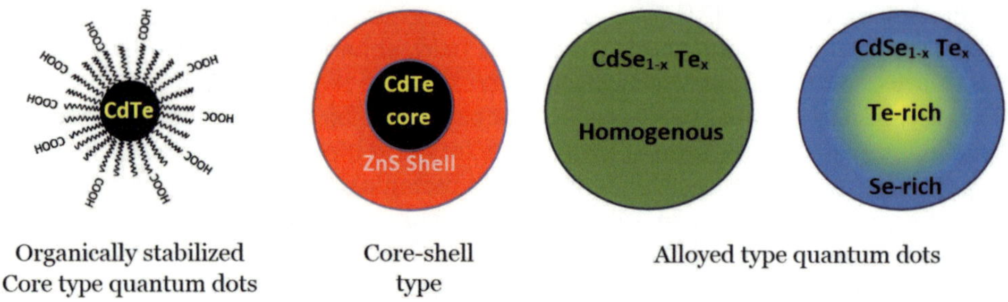


**Figure 1.**
*Types of quantum dots used in drug delivery [44].*

Core-shell-type quantum dots, such as CdTe/CdSe [41], CdSe/ZnS [42], CdSe/CdS, etc., are comprised of an inorganic core and an inorganic shell, generally a higher bandgap semiconductor around the core. Core-shell structures of quantum dots are more effective and have an intense brightness, as a result of the diminished chemical damage that can be happened to the fluorescence core. It is believed that inorganic core-shell quantum dots are more robust than organically passivated core-type quantum dots [43].

Alloyed quantum dots are synthesized by alloying two semiconductors with different bandgap energies. This type emits colors by just altering the composition rather than changing the crystallite size as a result of both homogenous and gradient internal structures [44].

### *2.2.2 Synthesis of quantum dots*

Among several methods utilized to synthesis quantum dots, hydrothermal synthesis [45, 46], and organometallic synthesis [47, 48] are the mainly used two techniques. Other methods, for instance, polyol-hydrolysis [49], electron beam irradiation [50], microwave-assisted aqueous synthesis [51], photochemical synthesis [52], UV irradiation [53], and chemical precipitation [54], are also less commonly used for quantum dot synthesis. CdTe quantum dots are highly used in biomedical applications compared to other types of quantum dots. Generally, CdTe quantum dots demonstrate inferior biocompatibility and stability in biological systems. Therefore, methods have developed to modify the surface of CdTe quantum dots during synthesis by capping the quantum dots using different stabilizers such as trioctylphosphine (TOP)/trioctylphosphine oxide (TOPO) [55], etc. Particularly, quantum dots which are capped with stabilizers containing thiol groups [56] make the quantum dots highly biocompatible and more stable inside biological environment [57, 58]. The CdTe quantum dots, which are synthesized in aqueous medium using thioglycolic acid [59], cysteine [60], and glutathione [61], provide high luminescence, stability, and surface functionalization to conjugate biomolecules.

### *2.2.3 Biomedical application*

Recently, quantum dots are used in many biotechnological appliances [6, 62]. These fluorescent nanocrystals are utilized in many immunofluorescence assays [63], tissue engineering [64], DNA array technology [65], and other cell biology techniques [66] where fluorescence measurements are occupied. Single-molecule level studies of living cells [67] and targeted drug delivery for cancer treatment [68] are some other applications in medicine. There are many advantages of using quantum dots in biotechnology. As the fluorescence of quantum dots is intense than other conventional dyes classically used in immuno-labeling and staining of proteins, quantum dots are currently being used in immunoassays as fluorophores [69] and in immuno-staining of cells [70], DNA [71], etc.

## 3. Advantages and advances in encapsulation of nanoparticles for bioconjugation

Bare nanoparticles often show undesirable properties in biological systems. These nanoparticles are often hydrophobic or hydrophilic, susceptible to oxidation and agglomeration. The main concern with magnetic nanoparticles is that they may fail to exhibit their super-paramagnetic properties inside or when conjugated to biological systems. This reduction of magnetism occurs as a consequence of their high chemical reactivity and extraordinary surface energy [16]. With the intention of maintaining nanoparticles in the colloidal condition during storage and to increase their constancy and biocompatibility, bare nanoparticles are further modified. Generally, surface modification is performed using polymers or surfactants which are hefty or charged molecules compared to the nanoparticles. These modifications provide several advantages such as increased physical and chemical stability. Therefore, the agglomeration and oxidation which are the most problematic concerns in biomedical applications can be minimized or limited. Ultimately, these modifications make the nanoparticles biocompatible with enhanced surface activity. Following modifications, with the use of functional groups available on the surface of nanoparticles, targeted biomolecules can be anchored on nanoparticles [72]. Magnetic nanoparticles acquire higher surface energy due to its tremendous specific surface area of exposed atoms on its surface [73].

Simply, modification of magnetic nanoparticles can be achieved by surface coating of the nanoparticle with either organic or inorganic materials. Inorganic materials include silica [74] and carbon [74]. Silica is a widely used compound for surface modification of iron oxide nanoparticles. As a result of its low cytotoxicity, silica modified nanoparticles are considered as an excellent combination to be used in biological applications. Silica coatings provide reduced agglomeration along with enhanced stability which ultimately ensures biocompatible-modified magnetic nanoparticles [75]. Organic material coating involves the addition of the material on to the nanoparticle, and the surface structure of the nanoparticle is totally undisturbed. There are many organic materials used for this strategy. Some of them are dextran [76], chitosan [77], alginate [78], and polymers such as polyethylene glycol (PEG) [79], polyvinyl alcohol (PVA) [80], and polyvinylpyrrolidone (PVP) [81].

## 4. Different methods of drug delivery

In drug delivery systems and diagnostics, nanotechnology has become a leader in the current decade. Since the 1980s there has been a considerable number of research on using nanotechnology in drug delivery systems [82, 83]. Due to its unique properties, such as smaller nanoscale size, magnetism, and fluorescence, nanotechnology-based drug delivery systems have defeated the problems and barriers of drug therapy in the pharmaceutical industry. Studies demonstrate many nanoparticulate drug careers, namely, liposomes [84], microemulsions [85], nano-suspensions [86], and nanoparticles [87]. These can be administrated through parenteral, tablets, capsules (as hard gelatin or soft gelatin), and as oral liquid [88].

These nanoparticles are extraordinary carriers for drug delivery for cancer treatment since they are not uptaken by phagocytosis by the immune system due to its nanoscale size [89].

Nanotechnology-based drug delivery has now come into a point where it has developed a smart drug delivery system. The theory behind smart drug delivery technique is, when the nanoparticle system is provoked by biological, chemical, or physical stimuli (biomolecules, pH, light, temperature, etc.), physicochemical properties of nanoparticle system change rapidly [90]. These smart drug delivery systems can be programmed to release drugs according to the stimuli, and the flow rate of drug release can be regulated according to the environmental condition. It can also predict the drugs required and switch on and off the release of drugs [91]. These advances have made the system more effective and have reduced the toxicity and side effects of the nanoparticulate drug admonition.

## 4.1 Types of drug delivery

There are several drug delivery methods such as oral method [92], injection-based method [93], transdermal delivery [94], pulmonary drug delivery [95], and carrier-based method [96].

In oral drug delivery, formulations used in oral drug administration range from simple tablets to modified control release tablets. This involves the use of various polymers and hydrogel-based formulations [92]. Injection-based drug delivery provides fast systemic effects bypassing first pass metabolism. Using this method, the drugs can be administered in unconscious or comatose patients, and drugs having short half-life can also be infused continuously [93]. Pulmonary drug delivery involves the administration of drugs by inhalation through the mouth or nose. The alveolar epithelial gets contacted with the drugs, and this provides a good surface especially for lipid-soluble drugs [95]. In transdermal drug administration, adhesive patches containing the drugs are applied on the skin. The drugs pass the skin surface by diffusion and enter the systemic circulation by percutaneous absorption [94]. Carrier-based drug delivery is a novel method which has been experimenting over decades in order to escalate the efficiency and diminish the detrimental side effects of carrier systems. This method serves improved selectivity, effectiveness, and safety of drug administration [96].

### *4.1.1 Carrier-based drug delivery systems*

Carrier-based drug delivery system utilizes several carriers such as liposomes, microemulsions, micellar systems, aquasomes, and nanoparticles.

Liposomes are drug carriers with a spherical structure, constructed from one or several amphiphilic phospholipids and cholesterols. Using liposomes as vehicles in drug delivery provides various conveniences compared to other systems. These carriers are created as small structures (80–100 nm), with bilayers of phospholipids and cholesterols with an aqueous interior. As a result, lipophilic drugs can be encapsulated in the lipid bilayer and hydrophilic drugs in the aqueous interior [85]. Using liposomes are considered as a low-toxic method with minimal side effects, and the drug can be applied without deteriorating its performance [84].

Microemulsions are a thermodynamically stable mixture of two immiscible liquids consisting of two phases called dispersed and continuous phase. These mixtures are typically stabilized with a surfactant and may have droplets with a size of 5–100 nm length [85]. Similar to emulsions, microemulsions can also be constructed as water in oil or oil in water. In drug administration, dispersed or continuous phases are determined by the hydrophilicity of the drug. Microemulsions provide increased solubility and stability of drugs enhancing high absorption rate through biological membranes.

Composed of copolymers and amphiphilic macromolecules with distinct hydrophobic and hydrophilic properties, polymer micelles form nanoscopic supramolecular core-shell structures. These structures show different types of morphologies, such as spheres, rods, vesicles, tubules, and lamellae. Core-shell structure of these particles grants a number of positive factors to be used in drug delivery applications [85]. As a result of the copolymers used in the formation of the micelles, the half-life of the system is expanded. Another consideration is that water-insoluble drugs can be solubilized by encapsulating the drug within the core structure. Due to its nanoscopic size, the permeability is intensified making it convenient for injections [97].

Aquasomes are spherical particles with 60–300 nm in size. These are used as vehicles for drug delivery as well as to deliver antigens to evoke antigen-specific immune responses [85]. These nanoparticles are comprised of a nanocrystalline core, which is responsible for the structural stability, and an oligomer coating, which protects the system from dehydration. As shown in **Figure 2**, the drugs or biomolecules of interest are adsorbed on the oligomeric coating of the aquasomes, making them conducive for drug delivery [98].

Nanoparticles are solid colloidal particles with 1–1000 nm size [18]. Currently, a number of different types of nanoparticles along with various macromolecules are used for drug delivery. Nanoparticles in different structures are produced depending on their configuration and utility such as nanotubes [99], nanowires [100], nanoshells [101], quantum dots [102], nanopores, nanobots [103], nano-erythrocytes [104], etc. Drugs or biomolecules are attached to the nanoparticles by adsorption, covalent attachment, or entrapment [18]. To be included in the drug development process, utilization of potentially toxic compounds or organic solvents in the nanoparticle synthesis procedure is inadvisable [44]. The components used in synthesis should ideally be biodegradable and safe for in vivo use. Further, these complexes should not induce immunological responses, and also, these should be stable under storage conditions [105]. In drug delivery, magnetic nanoparticles are being used in several approaches. The first approach is localized drug delivery, where the magnetic nanoparticles attached to the appropriate drug and administered systemically. When the magnetic field is applied on the required site of the body, these drug-containing magnetic nanoparticles will accumulate on the diseased site, and the drugs will be released for treatment [106]. The second approach is the usage of an alternate magnetic field to generate heat by magnetic nanoparticles which are conjugated to drugs via thermos-liable linker molecules [107]. These magnetic nanoparticles have the ability to generate heat when an alternate magnetic field is focused on a diseased site. Thus, under the alternate magnetic field, these thermos-liable linkers get cleaved, releasing the drugs [108].

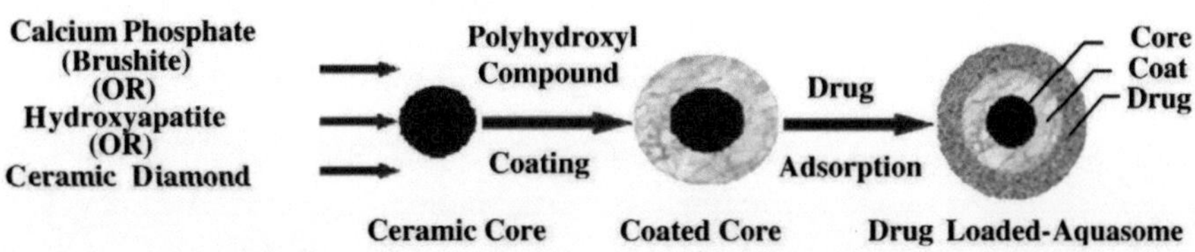


**Figure 2.**
*Preparation of aquasomes [98].*

## 5. Conclusion

Recent advances of nanotechnology which is used in biomedical science have given a great opportunity for the consumers to utilize the technology in a very efficient manner. Special focus on smart drug delivery technique which provides utmost advantages can prove this statement without hesitation. Nanoparticles, being considered as highly useful components in drug delivery, therapeutics, and diagnostics, can also affect its users negatively as a result of its inherent toxicity and inferior levels of biocompatibility. Even though different types of nanoparticles show diverse levels of toxicities, current appliances have made precautions to minimize its toxic effect and increase biocompatibility, by encapsulation. Magnetic nanoparticles and quantum dot nanoparticles, as discussed in this chapter, are used widely in the aforementioned applications with modified surface fabrications. The future prospects of nanotechnology in biomedical applications could lead to a highly sophisticated user-friendly technology where smarter appliances will reach consumers with the least challenges which they encounter in the present systems.

## Acknowledgements

Financial assistance given by the National Research Council, Sri Lanka (NRC-TO 14-04).

## Author details

Erandi Munasinghe[1]*, Maheshi Aththapaththu[2] and Lakmal Jayarathne[3]

1 Molecular Medicine Unit, Faculty of Medicine, University of Kelaniya, Sri Lanka

2 Biotechnology Unit, Industrial Technology Institute, Colombo, Sri Lanka

3 National Institute of Fundamental Studies, Kandy, Sri Lanka

*Address all correspondence to: erandieran@hotmail.com

## References

[1] Singh P, Pandit S, Mokkapati V, Garg A, Ravikumar V, Mijakovic I. Gold nanoparticles in diagnostics and therapeutics for human cancer. International Journal of Molecular Sciences. 2018;**19**(7):1979

[2] Dadfar SM, Roemhild K, Drude NI, von Stillfried S, Knüchel R, Kiessling F, et al. Iron oxide nanoparticles: Diagnostic, therapeutic and theranostic applications. Advanced Drug Delivery Reviews. 2019;**138**:302-325

[3] Manoharan K, Saha A, Bhattacharya S. Nanoparticles-based diagnostics. In: Environmental, Chemical and Medical Sensors. Singapore: Springer; 2018. pp. 253-269

[4] Khorram R, Raissi H, Morsali A, Shahabi M, et al. The computational study of the γ-Fe2O3 nanoparticle as carmustine drug delivery[PP3] system: DFT approach. Journal of Biomolecular Structure and Dynamics. 2019;**37**(2):454-464

[5] Gao W, Ji L, Li L, Cui G, Xu K, Li P, et al. Bifunctional combined Au-$Fe_2O_3$ nanoparticles for induction of cancer cell-specific apoptosis and real-time imaging. Biomaterials. 2012;**33**(14):3710-3718

[6] Qiu X, Hildebrandt N. Rapid and multiplexed microRNA diagnostic assay using quantum dot-based Forster resonance energy transfer. ACS Nano. 2015;**9**(8):8449-8457

[7] Bilan R, Nabiev I, Sukhanova A. Quantum dot-based Nanotools for bioimaging, diagnostics, and drug delivery. Chembiochem. 2016;**17**(22):2103-2114

[8] Zhang M, Wang W, Zhou N, Yuan P, Su Y, Shao M, et al. Near-infrared light triggered photo-therapy, in combination with chemotherapy using magnetofluorescent carbon quantum dots for effective cancer treating. Carbon. 2017;**118**:752-764

[9] Zhang D, Wei S, Kaila C, Su X, Wu J, Karki AB, et al. Carbon-stabilized iron nanoparticles for environmental remediation. Nanoscale. 2010;**2**(6):917-919

[10] Terris B, Thomson T. Nanofabricated and self-assembled magnetic structures as data storage media. Journal of Physics D: Applied Physics. 2005;**38**(12):R199

[11] Kefeni KK, Msagati TA, Mamba BB. Ferrite nanoparticles: Synthesis, characterisation and applications in electronic device. Materials Science and Engineering B. 2017;**215**:37-55

[12] Reddy LH, Arias JL, Nicolas J, Couvreur P. Magnetic nanoparticles: Design and characterization, toxicity and biocompatibility, pharmaceutical and biomedical applications. Chemical Reviews. 2012;**112**(11):5818-5878

[13] Nosrati H, Salehiabar M, Manjili HK, Danafar H, Davaran S. Preparation of magnetic albumin nanoparticles via a simple and one-pot desolvation and co-precipitation method for medical and pharmaceutical applications. International Journal of Biological Macromolecules. 2018;**108**:909-915

[14] Ahmad M, Minhas MU, Sohail M, Faisal M, Rashid H. Comprehensive review on magnetic drug delivery systems: A novel approach for drug targeting. Journal of Pharmacy and Alternative Medicine. 2013;**2**(4):13-21

[15] Katikaneani P, Vaddepally AK, Reddy Tippana N, Banavath R, Kommu S. Phase

transformation of iron oxide nanoparticles from hematite to maghemite in presence of polyethylene glycol: Application as corrosion resistant nanoparticle paints. Journal of Nanoscience. 2016. pp. 6

[16] Zhu N, Ji H, Yu P, Niu J, Farooq M, Akram M, et al. Surface modification of magnetic iron oxide nanoparticles. Nanomaterials. 2018;**8**(10):810

[17] Getzlaff M. Fundamentals of Magnetism. New York: Springer Science & Business Media; 2007

[18] Mathiyazhakan M, Xu C. Magnetic nanoparticles for drug delivery. In: Perspectives in Micro-and Nanotechnology for Biomedical Applications. Singapore: World Scientific; 2016. pp. 65-84

[19] Demangeat E, Pédrot M, Dia A, Bouhnik-Le-Coz M, Grasset F, Hanna K, et al. Colloidal and chemical stabilities of iron oxide nanoparticles in aqueous solutions: The interplay of structural, chemical and environmental drivers. Environmental Science: Nano. 2018;**5**(4):992-1001

[20] Sun S, Zeng H. Size-controlled synthesis of magnetite nanoparticles. Journal of the American Chemical Society. 2002;**124**(28):8204-8205

[21] Pankhurst QA, Connolly J, Jones S, Dobson J. Applications of magnetic nanoparticles in biomedicine. Journal of Physics D: Applied Physics. 2003;**36**(13):R167

[22] Liberti PA, Rao CG, Terstappen LW. Optimization of ferrofluids and protocols for the enrichment of breast tumor cells in blood. Journal of Magnetism and Magnetic Materials. 2001;**225**(1-2):301-307

[23] Inozemtseva OA, German SV, Navolokin NA, Bucharskaya AB, Maslyakova GN, Gorin DA. Encapsulated magnetite nanoparticles: Preparation and application as multifunctional tool for drug delivery systems. In: Nanotechnology and Biosensors. United Kingdom: Elsevier; 2018. pp. 175-192

[24] Cotin G, Perton F, Blanco-Andujar C, Pichon B, Mertz D, Bégin-Colin S. Design of anisotropic iron-oxide-based nanoparticles for magnetic hyperthermia. In: Nanomaterials for Magnetic and Optical Hyperthermia Applications. United Kingdom: Elsevier; 2019. pp. 41-60

[25] Sheng Y, Li S, Duan Z, Zhang R, Xue J. Fluorescent magnetic nanoparticles as minimally-invasive multi-functional theranostic platform for fluorescence imaging, MRI and magnetic hyperthermia. Materials Chemistry and Physics. 2018;**204**:388-396

[26] Xianyu Y, Wang Q, Chen Y. Magnetic particles-enabled biosensors for point-of-care testing. TrAC Trends in Analytical Chemistry. 2018;**106**:213-224

[27] Pöttler M, Fliedner A, Bergmann J, Bui LK, Mühlberger M, Braun C, et al. Magnetic tissue engineering of the vocal fold using superparamagnetic iron oxide nanoparticles. Tissue Engineering. 2019;Part A:25

[28] Kratz H, Taupitz M, de Schellenberger AA, Kosch O, Eberbeck D, Wagner S, et al. Novel magnetic multicore nanoparticles designed for MPI and other biomedical applications: From synthesis to first in vivo studies. PLoS One. 2018;**13**(1):e0190214

[29] Drbohlavova J, Adam V, Kizek R, Hubalek J. Quantum dots—Characterization, preparation and usage in biological systems. International Journal of Molecular Sciences. 2009;**10**(2):656-673

[30] Takagahara T, Takeda K. Theory of the quantum confinement effect on excitons in quantum dots of indirect-gap materials. Physical Review B. 1992;**46**(23):15578

[31] Lawandy NM. Quantum Dots, Semiconductor Nanocrystals and Semiconductor Particles used as Fluorescent Coding Elements; 2003, Google Patents

[32] William WY, Chang E, Drezek R, Colvin VL. Water-soluble quantum dots for biomedical applications. Biochemical and Biophysical Research Communications. 2006;**348**(3):781-786

[33] Hines DA, Kamat PV. Recent advances in quantum dot surface chemistry. ACS Applied Materials & Interfaces. 2014;**6**(5):3041-3057

[34] Christopoulos TK, Diamandis EP. Fluorescence immunoassays. In: Immunoassay. London: Elsevier; 1996. pp. 309-335

[35] Xu F, Kim HU, Kim J-H, Jung BJ, Grimsdale AC, Hwang D-H. Progress and perspective of iridium-containing phosphorescent polymers for light-emitting diodes. Progress in Polymer Science. 2015;**47**:92-121

[36] Liu F, Zhang Y, Ding C, Kobayashi S, Izuishi T, Nakazawa N, et al. Highly luminescent phase-stable CsPbI3 perovskite quantum dots achieving near 100% absolute photoluminescence quantum yield. ACS Nano. 2017;**11**(10):10373-10383

[37] Cui Q, Xu J, Wang X, Li L, Antonietti M, Shalom M. Phenyl-modified carbon nitride quantum dots with distinct photoluminescence behavior. Angewandte Chemie International Edition. 2016;**55**(11):3672-3676

[38] Lobo A, Möller T, Nagel M, Borchert H, Hickey SG, Weller H. Photoelectron spectroscopic investigations of chemical bonding in organically stabilized PbS nanocrystals. The Journal of Physical Chemistry B. 2005;**109**(37):17422-17428

[39] Vasudevan D, Gaddam RR, Trinchi A, Cole I. Core–shell quantum dots: Properties and applications. Journal of Alloys and Compounds. 2015;**636**:395-404

[40] Susumu K, Field LD, Oh E, Hunt M, Delehanty JB, Palomo V, et al. Purple-, blue-, and green-emitting multishell alloyed quantum dots: Synthesis, characterization, and application for ratiometric extracellular pH sensing. Chemistry of Materials. 2017;**29**(17):7330-7344

[41] Kim S, Fisher B, Eisler H-J, Bawendi M. Type-II quantum dots: CdTe/CdSe (core/shell) and CdSe/ZnTe (core/shell) heterostructures. Journal of the American Chemical Society. 2003;**125**(38):11466-11467

[42] Mathew S, Bhardwaj BS, Saran AD, Radhakrishnan P, Nampoori V, Vallabhan C, et al. Effect of ZnS shell on optical properties of CdSe–ZnS core–shell quantum dots. Optical Materials. 2015;**39**:46-51

[43] Dabbousi BO, Rodriguez-Viejo J, Mikulec FV, Heine JR, Mattoussi H, Ober R, et al. (CdSe) ZnS core–shell quantum dots: Synthesis and characterization of a size series of highly luminescent nanocrystallites. The Journal of Physical Chemistry B. 1997;**101**(46):9463-9475

[44] Bailey RE, Nie S. Alloyed semiconductor quantum dots: Tuning the optical properties without changing the particle size. Journal of the American Chemical Society. 2003;**125**(23):7100-7106

[45] Gu W, Yan Y, Zhang C, Ding C, Xian Y. One-step synthesis of

water-soluble MoS2 quantum dots via a hydrothermal method as a fluorescent probe for hyaluronidase detection. ACS Applied Materials & Interfaces. 2016;**8**(18):11272-11279

[46] Ren X, Pang L, Zhang Y, Ren X, Fan H, Liu SF. One-step hydrothermal synthesis of monolayer MoS2 quantum dots for highly efficient electrocatalytic hydrogen evolution. Journal of Materials Chemistry A. 2015;**3**(20):10693-10697

[47] Chen N, He Y, Su Y, Li X, Huang Q, Wang H, et al. The cytotoxicity of cadmium-based quantum dots. Biomaterials. 2012;**33**(5):1238-1244

[48] Bao H, Lu Z, Cui X, Qiao Y, Guo J, Anderson JM, et al. Extracellular microbial synthesis of biocompatible CdTe quantum dots. Acta Biomaterialia. 2010;**6**(9):3534-3541

[49] Xin Y, Yang X, Jiang P, Zhang Z, Wang Z, Zhang Y. Synthesis of CeO2-based quantum dots through a Polyol-hydrolysis method for fuel-borne catalysts. ChemCatChem. 2011;**3**(11):1772-1778

[50] Wang L, Li W, Wu B, Li Z, Pan D, Wu M. Room-temperature synthesis of graphene quantum dots via electron-beam irradiation and their application in cell imaging. Chemical Engineering Journal. 2017;**309**:374-380

[51] Zhang J, Chen Q, Zhang W, Mei S, He L, Zhu J, et al. Microwave-assisted aqueous synthesis of transition metal ions doped ZnSe/ZnS core/shell quantum dots with tunable white-light emission. Applied Surface Science. 2015;**351**:655-661

[52] Fageria P, Uppala S, Nazir R, Gangopadhyay S, Chang C-H, Basu M, et al. Synthesis of monometallic (Au and Pd) and bimetallic (AuPd) nanoparticles using carbon nitride (C3N4) quantum dots via the photochemical route for nitrophenol reduction. Langmuir. 2016;**32**(39):10054-10064

[53] Lu X, Wang R, Hao L, Yang F, Jiao W, Zhang J, et al. Preparation of quantum dots from MoO 3 nanosheets by UV irradiation and insight into morphology changes. Journal of Materials Chemistry C. 2016;**4**(48):11449-11456

[54] Rajabi HR, Farsi M. Study of capping agent effect on the structural, optical and photocatalytic properties of zinc sulfide quantum dots. Materials Science in Semiconductor Processing. 2016;**48**:14-22

[55] Paim APS, Rodrigues SSM, Ribeiro DS, de Souza GC, Santos JL, Araújo AN, et al. Fluorescence probe for mercury (ii) based on the aqueous synthesis of CdTe quantum dots stabilized with 2-mercaptoethanesulfonate. New Journal of Chemistry. 2017;**41**(9):3265-3272

[56] Wuister SF, de Mello Donega C, Meijerink A. Influence of thiol capping on the exciton luminescence and decay kinetics of CdTe and CdSe quantum dots. The Journal of Physical Chemistry B. 2004;**108**(45):17393-17397

[57] Wuister SF, Swart I, van Driel F, Hickey SG, de Mello Donegá C. Highly luminescent water-soluble CdTe quantum dots. Nano Letters. 2003;**3**(4):503-507

[58] Ma J, Chen J-Y, Guo J, Wang C, Yang W, Xu L, et al. Photostability of thiol-capped CdTe quantum dots in living cells: The effect of photo-oxidation. Nanotechnology. 2006;**17**(9):2083

[59] Jhonsi MA, Renganathan R. Investigations on the photoinduced interaction of water soluble thioglycolic acid (TGA) capped CdTe quantum dots with certain porphyrins. Journal

of Colloid and Interface Science. 2010;**344**(2):596-602

[60] Kim J, Huy BT, Sakthivel K, Choi HJ, Joo WH, Shin SK, et al. Highly fluorescent CdTe quantum dots with reduced cytotoxicity-a robust biomarker. Sensing and Bio-Sensing Research. 2015;**3**:46-52

[61] Zheng Y, Gao S, Ying JY. Synthesis and cell-imaging applications of glutathione-capped CdTe quantum dots. Advanced Materials. 2007;**19**(3):376-380

[62] Guo R, Zhou S, Li Y, Li X, Fan L, Voelcker NH. Rhodamine-functionalized graphene quantum dots for detection of Fe3+ in cancer stem cells. ACS Applied Materials & Interfaces. 2015;**7**(43):23958-23966

[63] Wu S, Liu L, Li G, Jing F, Mao H, Jin Q, et al. Multiplexed detection of lung cancer biomarkers based on quantum dots and microbeads. Talanta. 2016;**156**:48-54

[64] Zhao H, Ding R, Zhao X, Li Y, Qu L, Pei H, et al. Graphene-based nanomaterials for drug and/or gene delivery, bioimaging, and tissue engineering. Drug Discovery Today. 2017;**22**(9):1302-1317

[65] Fan L, Qi H, Teng J, Su B, Chen H, Wang C, et al. Identification of serum miRNAs by nano-quantum dots microarray as diagnostic biomarkers for early detection of non-small cell lung cancer. Tumor Biology. 2016;**37**(6):7777-7784

[66] Han H-S, Niemeyer E, Huang Y, Kamoun WS, Martin JD, Bhaumik J, et al. Quantum dot/antibody conjugates for in vivo cytometric imaging in mice. Proceedings of the National Academy of Sciences. 2015;**112**(5):1350-1355

[67] Baba K, Nishida K. Single-molecule tracking in living cells using single quantum dot applications. Theranostics. 2012;**2**(7):655

[68] Iannazzo D, Pistone A, Salamò M, Galvagno S, Romeo R, Giofré SV, et al. Graphene quantum dots for cancer targeted drug delivery. International Journal of Pharmaceutics. 2017;**518**(1-2):185-192

[69] Chen L, Yang G, Wu P, Cai C. Real-time fluorescence assay of alkaline phosphatase in living cells using boron-doped graphene quantum dots as fluorophores. Biosensors and Bioelectronics. 2017;**96**:294-299

[70] Tu C-C, Chen K-P, Yang T-A, Chou M-Y, Lin LY, Li Y-K. Silicon quantum dot nanoparticles with antifouling coatings for immunostaining on live cancer cells. ACS Applied Materials & Interfaces. 2016;**8**(22):13714-13723

[71] Wang G, Li Z, Ma N. Next-generation DNA-functionalized quantum dots as biological sensors. ACS Chemical Biology. 2017;**13**(7):1705-1713

[72] Jazayeri MH, Amani H, Pourfatollah AA, Pazoki-Toroudi H, Sedighimoghaddam B. Various methods of gold nanoparticles (GNPs) conjugation to antibodies. Sensing and Bio-Sensing Research. 2016;**9**:17-22

[73] Wu W, He Q, Jiang C. Magnetic iron oxide nanoparticles: Synthesis and surface functionalization strategies. Nanoscale Research Letters. 2008;**3**(11):397

[74] Yi DK, Selvan ST, Lee SS, Papaefthymiou GC, Kundaliya D, Ying JY. Silica-coated nanocomposites of magnetic nanoparticles and quantum dots. Journal of the American Chemical Society. 2005;**127**(14):4990-4991

[75] Malvindi MA, De Matteis V, Galeone A, Brunetti V, Anyfantis GC, Athanassiou A, et al. Toxicity assessment of silica coated

iron oxide nanoparticles and biocompatibility improvement by surface engineering. PLoS One. 2014;**9**(1):e85835

[76] Nath S, Kaittanis C, Ramachandran V, Dalal NS, Perez JM. Synthesis, magnetic characterization, and sensing applications of novel dextran-coated iron oxide nanorods. Chemistry of Materials. 2009;**21**(8):1761-1767

[77] Agnihotri SA, Mallikarjuna NN, Aminabhavi TM. Recent advances on chitosan-based micro-and nanoparticles in drug delivery. Journal of Controlled Release. 2004;**100**(1):5-28

[78] Castelló J, Gallardo M, Busquets MA, Estelrich J. Chitosan (or alginate)-coated iron oxide nanoparticles: A comparative study. Colloids and Surfaces A: Physicochemical and Engineering Aspects. 2015;**468**:151-158

[79] Inchaurraga L, Martín-Arbella N, Zabaleta V, Quincoces G, Peñuelas I, Irache JM. In vivo study of the mucus-permeating properties of PEG-coated nanoparticles following oral administration. European Journal of Pharmaceutics and Biopharmaceutics. 2015;**97**:280-289

[80] Strehl C, Schellmann S, Maurizi L, Hofmann-Amtenbrink M, Häupl T, Hofmann H, et al. Effects of PVA-coated nanoparticles on human T helper cell activity. Toxicology Letters. 2016;**245**:52-58

[81] Jaberolansar E, Kameli P, Ahmadvand H, Salamati H. Synthesis and characterization of PVP-coated Co0. 3Zn0. 7Fe2O4 ferrite nanoparticles. Journal of Magnetism and Magnetic Materials. 2016;**404**:21-28

[82] Labhasetwar V, Dorle A. Nanoparticles—A colloidal drug delivery system for primaquine and metronidazole. Journal of Controlled Release. 1990;**12**(2):113-119

[83] Li VH, Wood RW, Kreuter J, Harmia T, Robinson JR. Ocular drug delivery of progesterone using nanoparticles. Journal of Microencapsulation. 1986;**3**(3):213-218

[84] Malam Y, Loizidou M, Seifalian AM. Liposomes and nanoparticles: Nanosized vehicles for drug delivery in cancer. Trends in Pharmacological Sciences. 2009;**30**(11):592-599

[85] Majuru S, Oyewumi MO. Nanotechnology in drug development and life cycle management. In: Nanotechnology in Drug Delivery. New York: Springer; 2009. pp. 597-619

[86] Yadollahi R, Vasilev K, Simovic S. Nanosuspension technologies for delivery of poorly soluble drugs. Journal of Nanomaterials. 2015;**2015**:1

[87] Sahoo SK, Misra R, Parveen S. Nanoparticles: A boon to drug delivery, therapeutics, diagnostics and imaging. In: Nanomedicine in Cancer. Singapore: Pan Stanford; 2017. pp. 73-124

[88] De Villiers MM, Aramwit P, Kwon GS. Nanotechnology in Drug Delivery. New York: Springer Science & Business Media; 2008

[89] Zahr AS, de Villiers M, Pishko MV. Encapsulation of drug nanoparticles in self-assembled macromolecular nanoshells. Langmuir. 2005;**21**(1):403-410

[90] Liu D, Yang F, Xiong F, Gu N. The smart drug delivery system and its clinical potential. Theranostics. 2016;**6**(9):1306

[91] Cui W, Li J, Decher G. Self-assembled smart Nanocarriers for targeted drug delivery. Advanced Materials. 2016;**28**(6):1302-1311

[92] Amidon S, Brown JE, Dave VS. Colon-targeted oral drug delivery systems: Design trends and approaches. AAPS PharmSciTech. 2015;**16**(4):731-741

[93] Norouzi M, Nazari B, Miller DW. Injectable hydrogel-based drug delivery systems for local cancer therapy. Drug Discovery Today. 2016;**21**(11):1835-1849

[94] Marwah H, Garg T, Goyal AK, Rath G. Permeation enhancer strategies in transdermal drug delivery. Drug Delivery. 2016;**23**(2):564-578

[95] Pham D-D, Fattal E, Tsapis N. Pulmonary drug delivery systems for tuberculosis treatment. International Journal of Pharmaceutics. 2015;**478**(2):517-529

[96] Chen D, Lian S, Sun J, Liu Z, Zhao F, Jiang Y, et al. Design of novel multifunctional targeting nano-carrier drug delivery system based on CD44 receptor and tumor microenvironment pH condition. Drug Delivery. 2016;**23**(3):798-803

[97] Poelma SO, Oh SS, Helmy S, Knight AS, Burnett GL, Soh HT, et al. Controlled drug release to cancer cells from modular one-photon visible light-responsive micellar system. Chemical Communications. 2016;**52**(69):10525-10528

[98] Umashankar MS, Sachdeva RK, Gulati M. Aquasomes: A promising carrier for peptides and protein delivery. Nanomedicine: Nanotechnology, Biology and Medicine. 2010;**6**(3):419-426

[99] Bianco A, Kostarelos K, Prato M. Applications of carbon nanotubes in drug delivery. Current Opinion in Chemical Biology. 2005;**9**(6):674-679

[100] Pondman KM, Bunt ND, Maijenburg AW, van Wezel RJ, Kishore U, Abelmann L, et al. Magnetic drug delivery with FePd nanowires. Journal of Magnetism and Magnetic Materials. 2015;**380**:299-306

[101] Lee S-Y, Shieh M-J. Combined photothermo-chemotherapy using gold nanoshells on drug-loaded micelles for colorectal cancer treatment. In: Colloidal Nanoparticles for Biomedical Applications XIII. California, United States: International Society for Optics and Photonics; 2018

[102] Iannazzo D, Pistone A, Celesti C, Triolo C, Patané S, Giofré SV, et al. A smart Nanovector for cancer targeted drug delivery based on Graphene quantum dots. Nanomaterials. 2019;**9**(2):282

[103] Hortelão AC, Patiño T, Perez-Jiménez A, Blanco À, Sánchez S. Enzyme-powered Nanobots enhance anticancer drug delivery. Advanced Functional Materials. 2018;**28**(25):1705086

[104] Hu CMJ, Fang RH, Zhang L. Erythrocyte-inspired delivery systems. Advanced Healthcare Materials. 2012;**1**(5):537-547

[105] Tiwari G, Tiwari R, Sriwastawa B, Bhati L, Pandey S, Pandey P, et al. Drug delivery systems: An updated review. International Journal of Pharmaceutical Investigation. 2012;**2**(1):2

[106] Singh R, Lillard JW Jr. Nanoparticle-based targeted drug delivery. Experimental and Molecular Pathology. 2009;**86**(3):215-223

[107] Kim D-H, Nikles DE, Johnson DT, Brazel CS. Heat generation of aqueously dispersed CoFe2O4 nanoparticles as heating agents for magnetically activated drug delivery and hyperthermia. Journal of Magnetism and Magnetic Materials. 2008;**320**(19):2390-2396

[108] Kim S, Kwon K, Kwon IC, Park K. Nanotechnology in drug delivery: Past, present, and future. In: Nanotechnology in Drug Delivery. New York: Springer; 2009. pp. 581-596

Chapter 3

# Adsorption Configurations of 2-Chlorophenols on Colloidal Silica

*Lakmal Jayarathna, Nelum Karunathilake, Athula Bandara and Rohan Weerasooriya*

## Abstract

Chlorophenol (CP) is the organic-chloride compound which widely used as pesticides. Industrialization and modern agriculture release a vast amount of chlorophenol to the environment. Adsorption behavior and retention of chlorophenol in the environment still not cleared. Interaction of 2-chlorophenol (2-CP) with silica surface was investigated with different reaction conditions. The study was conformed that outer-sphere complexation of 2-CP with silica surface and different surface speciation was observed at different pH conditions. Maximum adsorption ($1.5 \times 10^{-8}$ mol $m^{-2}$) was observed around neutral pH conditions. 2-CP adsorption on silica surface followed the first order kinetics, and it indicates multilayer formation through capillary condensation. FTIR spectral analysis reveals the formation of a bidentate complex on the silica surface with 2-CP.

**Keywords:** adsorption, chlorophenol, complexation, FTIR, silica

## 1. Introduction

Industrialization and sophisticated agricultural techniques discharge many chlorinated compounds into the environment as primary organic pollutants [1]. Chlorophenols (CP) is designated as the most toxic organic pollutants in the list of hazardous wastes since these have a strong resistance to physical, chemical, or biological treatments [2, 3]. CPs have been used in agriculture, industry, and public health since 1920s [2]. Uses of malathion introduce 2-chlorophenol (2-CP) to the environment as one of the main toxic organic pollutant [4, 5].

2-CP is toxic, resistant to microbial attack, and accumulates in the food chain even from chlorophenol treated materials [6]. Accidental spillage, misuse, and improper disposal have resulted in ground water pollution [6, 7].

2-CP is lethal to a variety of organisms at the level of 1 mg $dm^{-3}$ [8]. Direct exposure of 2-CP is fatal, and the long term exposure of 2-CP may cause cancers and affect the function of the liver and immune system [3].

Although the production and the use of these are banned in some countries, chlorophenols are found in many parts of the world due to abundant usage and their environmental transportation. Owing to the toxicity and persistence of chlorophenol the controlling its levels and reducing the diffusion in the environment is necessary. In literature, the standard concentration levels for chlorophenols in industrial effluent and waters is set to 2 and 0.1 μg $L^{-1}$, respectively [9].

The fate and the diffusion of CPs depend on the neutral and ionic forms (speciation) of them. pH value of the aqueous phase governs the partition of the CP between different environments. Neutral form of CPs exhibit low solubility in water and high sorption capacity in soils, whereas the ionic form of CPs enhances the solubility in water and mobility in aqueous phase [10].

Adsorption is the major technique used for the removal or reduction of chlorinated compounds. Clays have been widely used as adsorbent due to their high specific surface area [10]. There are several reports appeared in the literature on the usage of different clay minerals as an absorbent for the removal of chlorinated pollutants [11]. These studies have proven to be very useful in describing the macroscopic nature of adsorption and adsorption kinetics. *In-situ* spectroscopic measurements further provide information on the adsorbate configurations and possible intermediates involved in some surface mediated reactions [12]. The stability of adsorbate's configuration and intermediates depends on numerous factors such as the structure of the surface and a complex formed, the coordination number of the metal atom in the complex, the thermodynamic equilibrium constant of the reaction, pH of the medium, etc. [13].

Surface properties of the adsorbents play central role in the adsorption process. The porosity of the surface and functional groups present on the surface are the main factors that govern the adsorption process [14, 15]. The efficiency of the clay mineral in the adsorption has been thoroughly investigated by several researchers [16]. Functional groups present in the organic compounds or the charge of the metal ions interest favorably with the specific properties of the mineral to enhance the adsorption. The adsorption process is influenced by many factors such as the chemical form of the adsorbate, solution pH, time of contact, adsorbate concentration, the amount of adsorbent, particle size, presence of competing adsorbates and others [17, 18].

Adsorption is one complex process involves in clay minerals with the association of contaminants. It is a mass transfer process from the aqueous phase to the solid phase accompanied by chemical and physical forces [19]. Physical characteristics of clay minerals are the governing factors in the adsorption process. Silica is reported as popular model adsorbent in the adsorption studies as it is the major constituent of natural clays by restricting the adsorption on one component. Low cost, non-toxicity, and the structural arrangements of them favor the adsorption of toxic contaminants. Silica is used as a model of soil adsorbent due to prevalence in the environment and well-characterized surface properties. The surface area of silica is an essential factor because the extent of the available surface is correlated with the surface reactivity [20].

The objective of this research is to investigate the adsorption behavior and configurations of 2-CP with silica surface using UV-visible and FT-IR spectroscopic methods.

## 2. Materials and methods

Colloidal silica was obtained from Fluka (Switzerland). All the other chemicals were purchased from Sigma Aldrich. Stock solutions of 2-CP and 20 g $dm^{-3}$ suspension of silica were prepared in deionized water. The suspension was stirred for 12 hours for equilibrating. The ionic strength of the suspensions was varied in the range of 0.0001–0.01 mol $dm^{-3}$ using 0.10 mol $dm^{-3}$ $NaNO_3$ solutions. All experiments were repeated for silicate suspensions with different ionic strength conditions.

An aliquot of silica suspensions was pipetted out to Duran 100 mL sealed type laboratory glass bottle and initial solution pH values were adjusted in the pH range from 2 to 12. Known amount of 2-CP was added to silicate suspensions. Then the system was sealed and was stirred for 1 hour. The final concentration of 2-CP was determined. The effect of the initial concentration of 2-CP and effect of contact time was studied.

The treated solid silica sample was recovered after the centrifugation and used for the FT-IR measurements after subsequent dying for appropriate times to eliminate water from samples. FT-IR measurements were carried out using JASCO FT-IR 410 spectrometer.

## 3. Results and discussion

### 3.1 Effect of pH and ionic strength

Variation of the adsorption density with pH is shown in the **Figure 1**. Similar pattern was observed at different ionic strength conditions.

When examining the values of initial and final pH, initial pH was higher than the final pH after adsorption under acidic condition and vice-versa under basic condition. Therefore, it will predict the different types of surface interactions between 2-CP and hydroxyl groups present on silica which are responsible for the changing in solution pH due to the adsorption process [20–22].

Under the acidic conditions, 2-CP interacts with surface silanol groups releasing $-H_2O$ molecule to the medium resulting increase the final pH [20]. Surface interactions between 2-CP and silanol groups in the acidic condition are shown in **Figure 2**.

The surface interactions between silanols and 2-CP under basic conditions are shown in **Figure 3**. Decrease of final solution pH is due to the releasing of $-HCl$ molecule to the medium by forming a bi-dentate diphenolate complex. This observation further conformed by spectroscopic studies.

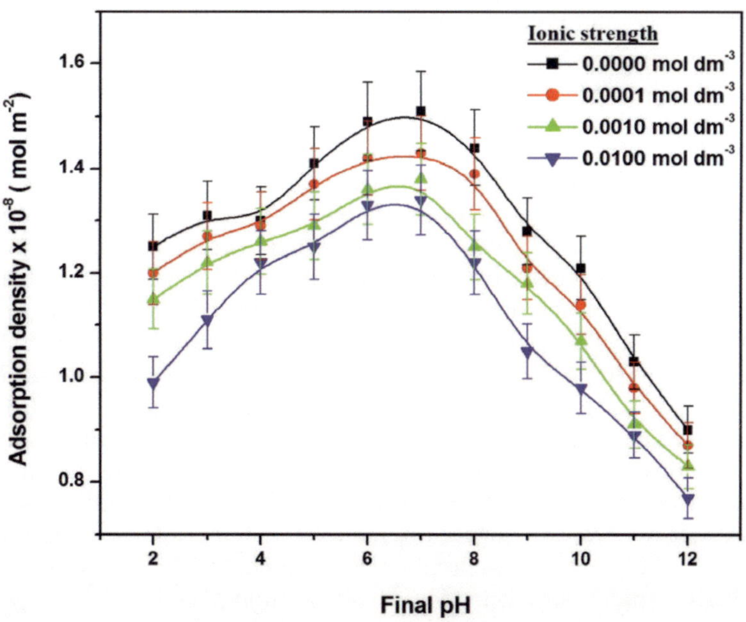


**Figure 1.**
*Adsorption density of 2-CP as a function of initial pH with different background ionic strength conditions with $NaNO_3$.*

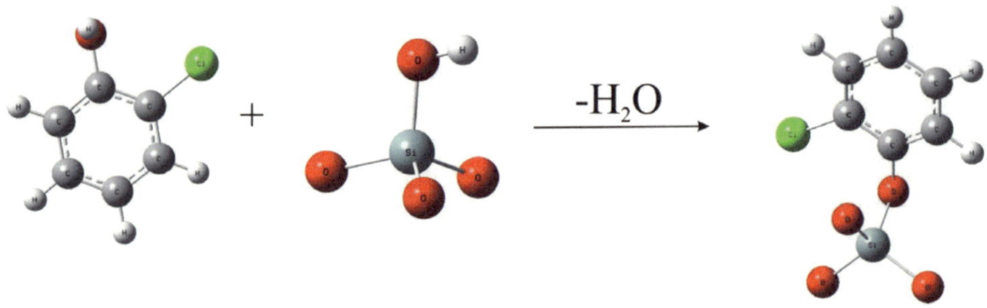


**Figure 2.**
*Proposed surface complexation of 2-CP with silica surface at acidic conditions.*

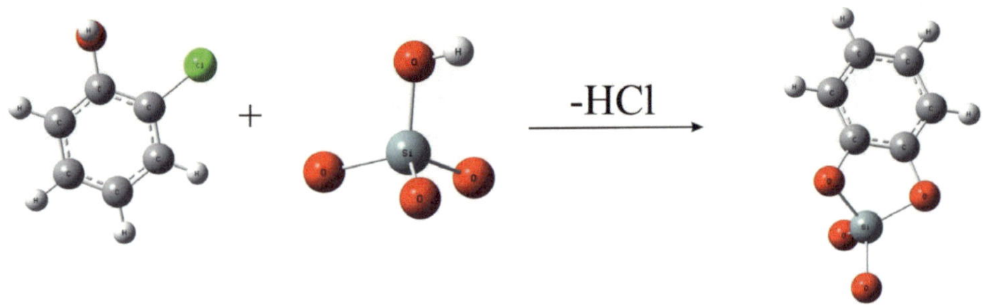


**Figure 3.**
*Proposed surface complexation of 2-CP with silica surface at basic conditions.*

According to **Figure 1**, the adsorption density increased significantly from pH 2 to 7 and then decreased gradually solution pH up to 12. The maximum adsorption capacity was observed around pH 7.

Experimental results revealed that surface charge of the species present in the system at different pH conditions governs the surface interactions between the silica and adsorbate, resulting in variation in adsorption densities [23]. Further, the important parameters such as dissociation constant and the point of zero charges of adsorbent affect the adsorption amount [18]. Point of zero charge ($pH_{ZPC}$) of silica is 3.5 [24]. Surface charge of silica is positive below the $pH_{ZPC}$ and negative above the $pH_{ZPC}$. Dissociation constant ($pK_a$) of 2-CP is 8.10 [25–27].

According to the $pK_a$ value, 2-CP dissociated into negative charge ions over the pH range of 9–12, and it remains as neutral molecule in the pH range of 2–7.8. Further, most of the silanol groups were neutral around pH 6. Dominant silanol groups were positively charged in the pH range of 2–3 and negatively charged in the pH range of 8–12.

The dissociation of 2-CP showed a negative effect on the adsorption mechanism due to the repulsive forces between negatively charged silanol groups and 2-CP ion. Therefore, the adsorption amount was low in the pH range of 10–12. Surface interactions between the less number of undissociated 2-CP and silica molecules showed a significant amount of adsorption even under the extreme acidic and basic conditions. However, the adsorption density was higher in the acidic region than in the alkaline area because the surface interactions were feasible due to the absence of molecules. Favorable surface interactions between neutral 2-CP and silanol groups showed a higher amount of adsorption density around pH 6 [28].

Furthermore, according to **Figure 1**, it shows that adsorption density was inversely proportional to the ionic strength of the medium. Effect of ionic strength on the adsorption process indicated that adsorption on to variable charge mineral surfaces could form outer-sphere complexes via electrostatic interactions [20, 29].

Outer-sphere complexation is sensitive to the changes of ionic strength due to the competition with counter ions in the background electrolytes [30]. Competition between counter ions and adsorbate was more significant at higher ionic strength conditions than at lower ionic strength conditions. These facts prove the formation of outer-sphere complexes upon the adsorption of 2-CP on silica [30].

### 3.2 FTIR investigation

Adsorption configuration between surface silanols groups and 2-CP at different pH conditions further confirmed by FT-IR spectral studies. **Figure 4(a)** shows the FT-IR spectra of untreated silica along with the adsorbed 2-CP at different solution pH conditions. Spectrum is divided into two parts of 500–1800 $cm^{-1}$, and 2800–4000 $cm^{-1}$ for simplicity as no bands were observed between 1800 and 2800 $cm^{-1}$. The spectrum of untreated silica is shown in line (A).

In the spectrum A, the bands for Si-OH bending modes at ~1080–1270 $cm^{-1}$, Si-OH deformation mode at ~811 $cm^{-1}$ and Si-O stretching mode at ~915 $cm^{-1}$ were observed. In addition to these characteristic bands, a band appeared at ~1637 $cm^{-1}$ could be attributed to the H-O-H bending vibration of physically adsorbed water as the broad band further supports this at ~3475 $cm^{-1}$ [21, 31]. The band at 3743 $cm^{-1}$ is typical for isolated O-H stretching vibration, and it indicates that the presence of isolated OH groups on the surface [32]. It was observed that the adsorption of 2-CP onto silica surface influence the IR spectrum of the untreated silica. For better comparison, IR spectra of silica surface treated with 2-CP at pH 5 and 9 are shown in lines (B) and (C), respectively, in **Figure 4(a)**. These spectra were measured after 3 hour equilibration time of the silica with 2-CP at respective pH. Upon adsorption of 2-CP, new bands appeared at 1280, 1482 and ~3030–3070 $cm^{-1}$ with an observation of complete disappearance of the isolated O-H groups at 3743 $cm^{-1}$ while all the other bands of untreated silica showed significant losses in their intensities. These observations suggest that the 2-CP chemisorbed on the surface [33, 34]. This behavior of chemisorption is further explained in **Figure 4(b)** where the difference

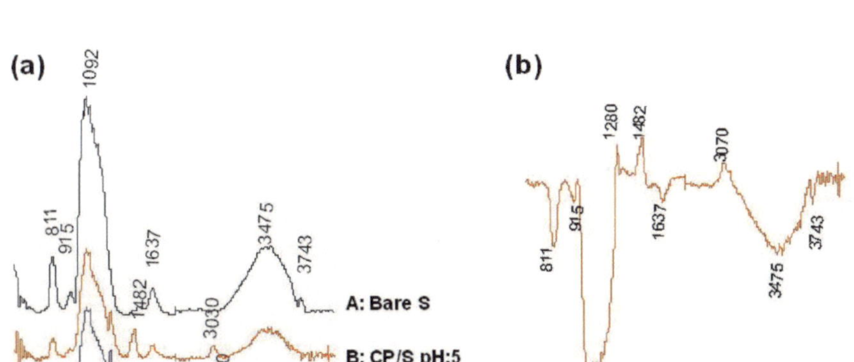


**Figure 4.**
*(a) FTIR spectra of (A) bare silica, (B) silica treated with 2-CP at pH 5 and (C) silica treated with 2-CP at pH 9. The bare silica samples prepare at pH 5 and 9 gave coincident spectra. All the spectra are plotted in the same scale for direct comparison. Scale is broken between 1800 and 2750 $cm^{-1}$ as no bands were observed in the region. (b) Difference spectrum at pH 9. The positive bands are characteristic for 2-CP on the surface while negative bands indicate the loss of surface sites due to chemisorption of 2-CP.*

spectrum (2-CP adsorbed—bare silica) is depicted. Negative bands at ~811, 915, 1270, 1637, 3475 and 3743 $cm^{-1}$ suggest the loss of original nature of Si-O(H) moieties upon adsorption of 2-CP while the positive bands appeared at ~1280, 1482 and 3070 $cm^{-1}$ clearly shows the presence of 2-CP on the surface [21]. The disappearance of 3743 $cm^{-1}$ bands indicated that the isolated hydroxyl groups are one of the major adsorption sites for 2-CP. Reduced intensities of other characteristic bands of silica further suggest the interaction of 2-CP with the surface. The new bands appeared at 1280, 1482 and 3050 $cm^{-1}$ are assigned to the C-O stretching, C=C stretching of the benzene ring, and aromatic C-H stretching modes, respectively, of 2-CP [31]. It should note here that the 1280 $cm^{-1}$ band appeared at pH 9 is more intense compared to that observed at pH 5 even though the amount adsorbed (64%) was lesser than that observed at pH 5 (74%) [33, 34].

The IR observations can further explain the variation of solution pH with the adsorption. **Figure 5(a)** shows the results in the 1400–1800 $cm^{-1}$ region for the untreated (bare: dash-dot line) silica, and silica treated with 2-CP at pH 5 (line A) and 9 (line B).

As described earlier, the intensity of the band due to H-O-H bending mode of silica at 1637 $cm^{-1}$ decreased in intensity and shifted to around 1630 $cm^{-1}$ upon adsorption of 2-CP in both cases. When the pH of the medium was 9, the band at 1637 $cm^{-1}$ lost its intensity with the appearance of a new band at 1607 $cm^{-1}$. Also, a clear change was observed in the band at ~1482 $cm^{-1}$. A new band appeared at 1495 $cm^{-1}$ with a remaining shoulder at ~1477 $cm^{-1}$ and a second shoulder at ~1452 $cm^{-1}$ was observed. These observations suggest that different type of bonding species are involved in these two pH conditions. The new band appeared at 1495 $cm^{-1}$ along with the shift in the band at 1637–1607 $cm^{-1}$ reveal the formation of catechol type intermediate [35, 36]. The bands at 1495 $cm^{-1}$ can be attributed to the C-C stretch of the above catechol type intermediate and that the appearance of strong band at 1280 $cm^{-1}$(**Figure 4**, line C) might indicate the presence of more-oriented C-O bonding in the same species of the above. The shift in 1482 $cm^{-1}$ band

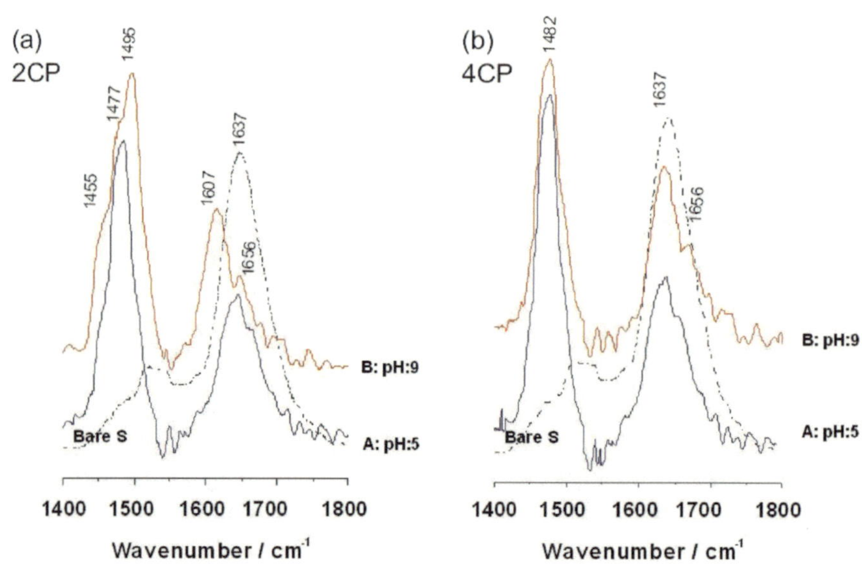


**Figure 5.**
*FTIR spectra in 1400–1800 $cm^{-1}$ region (a) 2-CP and (b) 4-CP, bare silica: dashed-dot line, (A) silica treated with 2 and 4 CP at pH 5 and (B) silica treated with 2 and 4 CPs at pH 9. The bare silica samples prepare at pH 5 and 9 gave coincident spectra. All the spectra are plotted in the same scale for direct comparison.*

to 1477 $cm^{-1}$ and another shoulder peak at ~455 $cm^{-1}$ indicate the changes in the electronic environment of the benzene ring due to the formation of catechol intermediate in which that can be in bi-dentate or bridging configuration to the silica surface. The experiments done with 4-CP further confirmed the formation of this intermediate and the results are shown in **Figure 5(b)**. The adsorption of 4-CPon silica at different pHs showed quite similar spectra and the bands at 1607 and 1495 $cm^{-1}$ did not appear. Further, the band shift at 1637 $cm^{-1}$ was negligible. 4-CP cannot form catechol type intermediate upon adsorption hence giving no bands around the above frequencies. Study on the adsorption of 2-CP vapor on fused silica at high temperature revealed that the formation of catechol type intermediate species by the bonding of 2-CP via Cl atom and phenolic oxygen and formation of such species are proved by the observation of a band at ~1600 and 1494 $cm^{-1}$ [25, 35, 37].

Though the pH 9 of the medium is higher than pKa of 2-CP (8.52) the above observations clearly show the supportive information for the proposed adsorbed species. When the pH is higher than pKa, anionic species formed may have a high tendency towards interacting with silica by the elimination of $H_2O$ and HCl molecules [33]. However, previous studies on the adsorption of 2-CP on fly ash and Ca-montmorillonite showed the reduction in the adsorption capacity when the pH was higher than pKa where the dissociated organic molecules experience the repulsion from the negatively charged surface [38]. In the present study, the amount adsorbed at pH 5 was ~74% while that at pH 9 was 64%. Despite that repulsion and ~10% reduction in the adsorption, the step of the elimination of Cl atom may make some favorable path for the remaining (or dissociated) 2-CP to interact with the Si-O sites [39].

## 4. Conclusions

Adsorption of 2-CP on silica surface was examined under different pH conditions. The maximum adsorption capacity of $1.5 \times 10^{-8}$ mol $m^{-2}$ on silica surface was observed at pH 7. There are different adsorbed species were predicted in different pH conditions. The interaction between colloidal silica ($SiO_2$) and 2-CP was investigated in an aqueous medium with the emphasis of Fourier Transform infrared (FT-IR) spectroscopy.

Effect of ionic strength on the adsorption was significant as the adsorption capacity was inversely proportional to the ionic strength of the medium. Experimental results confirmed the formation of outer-sphere complexes during the adsorption process. FTIR spectroscopic studies revealed the direct interaction between 2CP and silica via catechol type bidentate complex by eliminating HCl while the experiments with 4CP further confirmed the formation of such an adsorbate configuration. In the future, these observations can also apply to identify degradation pathways of 2-CP in natural soil system in different environmental conditions.

## Conflicts of interest

All the authors declare that there are no potential conflicts of interest in any financial or nonfinancial.

## Funding

This study was funded by National Institute of Fundamental Studies, Hanthana road, Kandy.

## Abbreviation

| | |
|---|---|
| 2-CP | 2-chlorophenol |

## Author details

Lakmal Jayarathna[1*], Nelum Karunathilake[2], Athula Bandara[3] and Rohan Weerasooriya[1]

1 National Institute of Fundamental Studies, Kandy, Sri Lanka

2 Postgraduate Institute of Science, University of Peradeniya, Peradeniya, Sri Lanka

3 Department of Chemistry, University of Peradeniya, Peradeniya, Sri Lanka

*Address all correspondence to: lakmalipj@yahoo.co.uk

## References

[1] Butter TJ, Evison LM, Hancock IC, Holland FS, Matis KA, Philipson A, et al. The removal and recovery of cadmium from dilute aqueous solutions by biosorption and electrolysis at laboratory scale. Water Research. 1998;**32**(2):400-406. DOI: 10.1016/S0043-1354(97)00273-X

[2] Zheng S, Yang Z, Jo DH, Park YH. Removal of chlorophenols from groundwater by chitosan sorption. Water Research. 2004;**38**(9):2315-2322. DOI: 10.1016/j.watres.2004.02.010

[3] Yu J-Y, Shin M-Y, Noh J-H, Seo J-J. Adsorption of phenol and chlorophenols on hexadecyltrimethylammonium- and tetramethylammonium-montmorillonite from aqueous solutions. Geosciences Journal. 2004;**8**(2):191. DOI: 10.1007/bf02910195

[4] Lacorte S, Viana P, Guillamon M, Tauler R, Vinhas T, Barcelo D. Main findings and conclusions of the implementation of directive 76/464/CEE concerning the monitoring of organic pollutants in surface waters (Portugal, April 1999-May 2000). Journal of Environmental Monitoring. 2001;**3**(5):475-482. DOI: 10.1039/b104832p

[5] Zhou L-C, Meng X-G, Fu J-W, Yang Y-C, Yang P, Mi C. Highly efficient adsorption of chlorophenols onto chemically modified chitosan. Applied Surface Science. 2014;**292**:735-741. DOI: 10.1016/j.apsusc.2013.12.041

[6] Edgehill RU, Finn RK. Isolation, characterization and growth kinetics of bacteria metabolizing pentachlorophenol. European Journal of Applied Microbiology and Biotechnology. 1982;**16**(4):179-184. DOI: 10.1007/bf00505829

[7] Yousef RI, El-Eswed B. The effect of pH on the adsorption of phenol and chlorophenols onto natural zeolite. Colloids and Surfaces A: Physicochemical and Engineering Aspects. 2009;**334**(1):92-99. DOI: 10.1016/j.colsurfa.2008.10.004

[8] Gonzalez JF, Hu W-S. Effect of glutamate on the degradation of pentachlorophenol by *Flavobacterium* sp. Applied Microbiology and Biotechnology. 1991;**35**(1):100-104. DOI: 10.1007/bf00180644

[9] Bazrafshan E, Mostafapour FK, Jafari Mansourian H. Phenolic compounds: Health effects and its removal from aqueous environments by low cost adsorbents. Health Scope. 2013;**2**(2):65-66

[10] Murcia MD, Gomez M, Gomez E, Bodalo A, Gomez JL, Hidalgo AM. Assessing combination treatment, enzymatic oxidation and ultrafiltration in a membrane bioreactor, for 4-chlorophenol removal: Experimental and modeling. Journal of Membrane Science. 2009;**342**(1):198-207. DOI: 10.1016/j.memsci.2009.06.037

[11] Ali I, Asim M, Khan TA. Low cost adsorbents for the removal of organic pollutants from wastewater. Journal of Environmental Management. 2012;**113**:170-183. DOI: 10.1016/j.jenvman.2012.08.028

[12] Li J, Cui H, Song X, Zhang G, Wang X, Song Q, et al. Adsorption and intercalation of organic pollutants and heavy metal ions into MgAl-LDHs nanosheets with high capacity. RSC Advances. 2016;**6**(95):92402-92410. DOI: 10.1039/c6ra18783h

[13] Wang C, Ma R, Wu Q, Sun M, Wang Z. Magnetic porous carbon as an adsorbent for the enrichment of chlorophenols from water and

peach juice samples. Journal of Chromatography A. 2014;**1361**:60-66. DOI: 10.1016/j.chroma.2014.08.002

[14] Zhang X, Bai R. Mechanisms and kinetics of humic acid adsorption onto chitosan-coated granules. Journal of Colloid and Interface Science. 2003;**264**(1):30-38. DOI: 10.1016/S0021-9797(03)00393-X

[15] Farrah H, Pickering W. The sorption of lead and cadmium species by clay minerals. Australian Journal of Chemistry. 1977;**30**(7):1417-1422. DOI: 10.1071/CH9771417

[16] Feddal I, Ramdani A, Taleb S, Gaigneaux EM, Batis N, Ghaffour N. Adsorption capacity of methylene blue, an organic pollutant, by montmorillonite clay. Desalination and Water Treatment. 2014;**52**(13-15):2654-2661. DOI: 10.1080/19443994.2013.865566

[17] Johnson BB. Effect of pH, temperature, and concentration on the adsorption of cadmium on goethite. Environmental Science & Technology. 1990;**24**(1):112-118. DOI: 10.1021/es00071a014

[18] Jarvis SC, Jones LHP. The contents and sorption of cadmium in some agricultural soils of England and Wales. Journal of Soil Science. 1980;**31**(3): 469-479. DOI: 10.1111/j.1365-2389.1980.tb02096.x

[19] Weerasooriya R, Wickramarathne HUS, Dharmagunawardhane HA. Surface complexation modeling of fluoride adsorption onto kaolinite. Colloids and Surfaces A: Physicochemical and Engineering Aspects. 1998;**144**(1):267-273. DOI: 10.1016/S0927-7757(98)00646-3

[20] Sayari A, Hamoudi S, Yang Y. Applications of pore-expanded mesoporous silica. 1. Removal of heavy metal cations and organic pollutants from wastewater. Chemistry of Materials. 2005;**17**(1):212-216. DOI: 10.1021/cm048393e

[21] Zhang L, Zhang B, Wu T, Sun D, Li Y. Adsorption behavior and mechanism of chlorophenols onto organoclays in aqueous solution. Colloids and Surfaces A: Physicochemical and Engineering Aspects. 2015;**484**:118-129. DOI: 10.1016/j.colsurfa.2015.07.055

[22] Wahab HS, Bredow T, Aliwi SM. A computational study on the adsorption and ring cleavage of para-chlorophenol on anatase $TiO_2$ surface. Surface Science. 2009;**603**(4):664-669. DOI: 10.1016/j.susc.2009.01.001

[23] Vaishya RC, Gupta SK. Modelling arsenic(III) adsorption from water by sulfate-modified iron oxide-coated sand (SMIOCS). Journal of Chemical Technology & Biotechnology. 2003;**78**(1):73-80. DOI: 10.1002/jctb.745

[24] Cho GS, Lee D-H, Lim HM, Lee S-H, Kim C, Kim DS. Characterization of surface charge and zeta potential of colloidal silica prepared by various methods. Korean Journal of Chemical Engineering. 2014;**31**(11):2088-2093. DOI: 10.1007/s11814-014-0112-5

[25] Soltani T, Lee B-K. Mechanism of highly efficient adsorption of 2-chlorophenol onto ultrasonic graphene materials: Comparison and equilibrium. Journal of Colloid and Interface Science. 2016;**481**:168-180. DOI: 10.1016/j.jcis.2016.07.049

[26] Shirzad-Siboni M, Jafari S-J, Farrokhi M, Yang JK. Removal of phenol from aqueous solutions by activated red mud: Equilibrium and kinetics studies. Environmental Engineering Research. 2013;**18**(4):247-252. DOI: 10.4491/eer.2013.18.4.247

[27] Uchida M, Okuwaki A. UV-vis spectrophotometric determination of the dissociation constants for

monochlorophenols in aqueous solution at elevated temperatures. Journal of Solution Chemistry. 2003;**32**(1):19-39. DOI: 10.1023/a:1022980614320

[28] Ghaffari A, Tehrani MS, Husain SW, Anbia M, Azar PA. Adsorption of chlorophenols from aqueous solution over amino-modified ordered nanoporous silica materials. Journal of Nanostructure in Chemistry. 2014;**4**(3):114. DOI: 10.1007/s40097-014-0114-1

[29] Hayes KF, Papelis C, Leckie JO. Modeling ionic strength effects on anion adsorption at hydrous oxide/solution interfaces. Journal of Colloid and Interface Science. 1988;**125**(2):717-726. DOI: 10.1016/0021-9797(88)90039-2

[30] Cea M, Seaman JC, Jara AA, Mora ML, Diez MC. Describing chlorophenol sorption on variable-charge soil using the triple-layer model. Journal of Colloid and Interface Science. 2005;**292**(1):171-178. DOI: 10.1016/j.jcis.2005.05.074

[31] Li Y, Li X, Dong C, Li Y, Jin P, Qi J. Selective recognition and removal of chlorophenols from aqueous solution using molecularly imprinted polymer prepared by reversible addition-fragmentation chain transfer polymerization. Biosensors and Bioelectronics. 2009;**25**(2):306-312. DOI: 10.1016/j.bios.2009.07.001

[32] Song D, Li J, Cai Q. In situ diffuse reflectance FTIR study of CO adsorbed on a cobalt catalyst supported by silica with different pore sizes. The Journal of Physical Chemistry C. 2007;**111**(51):18970-18979. DOI: 10.1021/jp0751357

[33] Mosallanejad S, Dlugogorski BZ, Kennedy EM, Stockenhuber M. Adsorption of 2-chlorophenol on the surface of silica- and alumina-supported iron oxide: An FTIR and XPS study. ChemCatChem. 2017;**9**(3):481-491. DOI: 10.1002/cctc.201601069

[34] Alderman SL, Dellinger B. FTIR investigation of 2-chlorophenol chemisorption on a silica surface from 200 to 500°C. The Journal of Physical Chemistry A. 2005;**109**(34):7725-7731. DOI: 10.1021/jp051071t

[35] Bardakçı B. Monitoring of monochlorophenols adsorbed on metal (Cu and Zn) supported pumice by infrared spectroscopy. Environmental Monitoring and Assessment. 2009;**148**(1):353-357. DOI: 10.1007/s10661-008-0165-1

[36] Lochab B, Shukla S, Varma IK. Naturally occurring phenolic sources: Monomers and polymers. RSC Advances. 2014;**4**(42):21712-21752. DOI: 10.1039/c4ra00181h

[37] Bustos-Ramírez K, Barrera-Díaz CE, De Icaza-Herrera M, Martínez-Hernández AL, Natividad-Rangel R, Velasco-Santos C. 4-chlorophenol removal from water using graphite and graphene oxides as photocatalysts. Journal of Environmental Health Science and Engineering. 2015;**13**(1):33. DOI: 10.1186/s40201-015-0184-0

[38] Yu J-Y, Shin M-Y, Noh J-H, Seo J-J. Adsorption of phenol and chlorophenols on Ca-montmorillonite in aqueous solutions. Geosciences Journal. 2004;**8**(2):185-189. DOI: 10.1007/bf02910194

[39] Hamdaoui O, Naffrechoux E. Modeling of adsorption isotherms of phenol and chlorophenols onto granular activated carbon: Part I. Two-parameter models and equations allowing determination of thermodynamic parameters. Journal of Hazardous Materials. 2007;**147**(1):381-394. DOI: https://doi.org/10.1016/j.jhazmat.2007.01.021

## Section 2

# Colloid Science and Biotechnology

Chapter 4

# Colloid Stability Influences on the Biological Organization and Functions

*Camillo La Mesa and Gianfranco Risuleo*

## Abstract

It is common to entities having sizes in the nano/micro-scale range be that, real or bio-intended systems, to undergo the action of many different forces, imparting them colloid stability. Ubiquitary electrostatic contributions, sometimes dominant, may overlap with steric stabilization ones; their combination effectively takes place in most cases. The two effects are jointly responsible, for instance, for the control of many phenomena such as: adhesion onto cells of alien agents, cellular separation during morpho-functional evolution, uptake of exogenous materials into cells and tissues. We evidence here, how the combination of these forces operates, and indicate the procedures leading to their effectiveness, when required for purposes inherent to biomimicry.

**Keywords:** biological systems, biomimetic systems, surface charge density, sterical stabilization, adhesion

## 1. Introduction

It took a long time before the characteristics peculiar to biological organisms, were considered on the more solid grounds dictated by Physics and Chemistry. It is enough to remind the violent criticism raised by many outstanding scientists against D'Arcy Thompson book "*On growth and form*", dating the second decade of the last century. The successful fate of the book urged biologists to account not only for the taxonomic rules inherent to biological organisms and to focus, much more reasonably, on the physical forces, geometrical, and morphological constraints responsible for biological organization, growth and functions. It is convincingly stated there that "In the growth of a shell, for instance, we can conceive no simpler law than this, that it shall widen and lengthen in the same unvarying proportions: and this simplest of laws is that which Nature tends to follow. The shell, like the creature within it, grows in size but does not change its shape; and the existence of this constant relativity of growth, or constant similarity of form, is of the essence, and may be made the basis of a definition, of the equiangular spiral." [1]. To the best of our knowledge this is the first effort to explain the growth of animal shapes in terms of geometry and topology, and to account for the modes in which organisms self-organize, following the rules dictated by their own genome. With respect to the gene/body shape one should consider the phenomenon of epistasis, i.e., the effect of one gene modulated by the genetic background [2]. Originally this definition meant that the phenotypic effect of one gene is affected by one or more different



IntechOpen

genetic *loci*. Thus, epistatic mutations have different "combinatorial" rather than individual effects. This was originally a genetics concept but, nowadays, is of common use in biochemistry, computational biology and evolutionary biology. Epistasis stems from interactions between or, reciprocally, within genes and this leads to non-linear effects. Therefore, it has a dramatic influence on the shape of evolutionary landscapes, which leads to profound consequences for evolution and evolutionary potentials of the phenotypic traits [3].

The statements of D'Arcy Thompson's statement become convincing also if applied to the micro/nanoscale range. Here, the role played by physical forces at short distances comes in full evidence, that is: when the biological organization modes in their lower stage, as in dispersed cells, are considered (however, in a fully organized, functional organism, the role of physical forces may become extremely complex). The stability and, eventually, the organization of such objects is dictated by the overlapping, or dominance, of van der Waals, *vdW*, electrostatic, osmotic, elastic, steric and many other forces. Their combination with what is dictated by gene expression, leads to an optimal topology-ruled shape that a biological system, be it a cell or a tissue, not to speak of a whole organism, assumes. In what follows we put in evidence the role of major contributions when the stabilization in dispersed form is required, or naturally occurs.

To proceed along this line, we discuss separately the physical origins of both electrostatic and steric effects. Examples based on real biological systems, shall be given and the pathways inducing/reducing the onset, or disappearance, of these effects will be discussed. We must be aware that the action of many forces is required to attain a preferred organization mode in cells and tissues, where electrostatic interactions are prevalent, safe the enzyme/substrate where VdW forces are prevalent. We also know that the mentioned forces are dominant, in the terms dictated by energy costs, not considering their modulus (provided the sum of all $\Delta G$ terms is $<0$). This fact, combined with the genetically driven rules, fulfills requirements needed for optimal biological activity and functions. In what follows we describe, in sequence, the quintessential features of both electrostatic and steric forces, which are required to understand how important they are in living systems. In the final part of this chapter we mention some pertinent examples on the role that electrostatic and steric effects may jointly play.

## 2. Electrostatic aspects

Sufficiently high electrical potentials, $\psi$, are responsible for the kinetic stability of colloids. These facts avoid the onset of undesired effects, such as sedimentation [4], creaming [5], and/or clustering [6]. The foundations of colloid stability date to the 1940s of the last century and are formalized in DLVO theory, which applies to real dispersions. The original theory combines electrostatics and statistical thermodynamics, and is formalized in the well-known Poisson-Boltzmann, or P-B, equation. The effects considered in that theory are responsible for the stabilization of clays [7], inorganic colloids as $Al(OH)_3$ [8], latexes [9], cells, vesicles, viruses, etc. [10–13]. Note that counter-ion condensation onto DNA, and biopolymers in general, is expressed in terms of the same theory [14, 15].

The balance of attractive vs. repulsive electrostatic forces depends on the sign of their surface potentials, $\psi$'s. On this line, Parsegian and Gingell showed that charged surfaces of the same sign, eventually differing in modulus, may never become attractive. Conversely, particles/surfaces bearing opposite sign attract or repel, depending on experimental conditions [16]. That statement was demonstrated for the surface charge densities of colloid *A* and *B*, termed $\sigma_A$ and $\sigma_B$, (with $\sigma_A \neq \sigma_B$)

separated by a distance $0 < x < l$. If the upper and lower limits of the derivative, hereafter indicated as $[d(ze\psi/KT)/dx]_{|x=0}$ and $[d(ze\psi/KT)/dx]_{|x=1}$, respectively, differ in sign, the corresponding function must be null somewhere between the integration limits. As a consequence, like-charged surfaces always repel, whatever is $x$, $\sigma$ or $\psi$. The question to be addressed is how to find rational procedures reducing that unescapable fate.

In what follows, we indicate how to face the problem and to control, or minimize, repulsions. Imagine having two large cells, each characterized by a given $\sigma$. We suppose that the respective surface charge densities are equal in modulus. The potential that one cell exerts on the other is $\psi$. In the P-B equation, the difference among the respective exponentials, that is, $\exp^{\pm(ze\psi/KT)}$, is considered. Proper transformation in hyperbolic form reduces the function to [17]

$$\exp^{+(ze\psi/KT)} - \exp^{-(ze\psi/KT)} = 2\sinh(ze\psi/KT) \tag{1}$$

which is easily linearized if $ze\psi << KT$. In words, the Euler-based approximation underlying Eq. (1) holds in linear perturbation regimes. The theory relies on the fact that the effect of $\psi$ decreases with distance from the source (i.e., where charges are located), and fulfills the law stating

$$\psi = \psi^o exp^{-kx} \tag{2}$$

Implicit in the equation is the statement that, a distance $x$ from a surface of well-defined potential, $\psi$ decreases and its decay depends on the number of charges; more properly, on the concentration in excess of positive, or negative, ions. In words, it is as if we were in presence of a double layer, of length $1/k$, located a distance $x$ apart from the source. To reduce the effect of $\psi$ on its surroundings, thus,

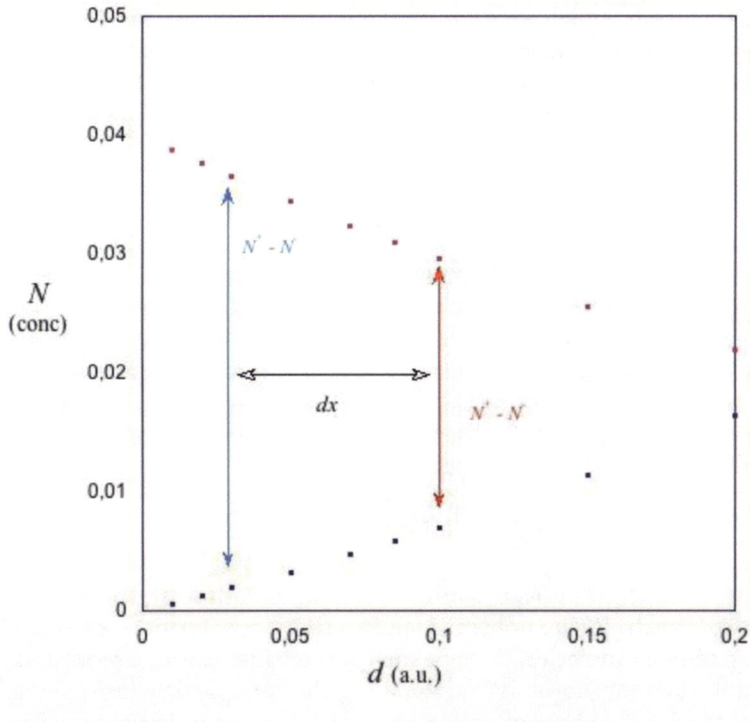


**Figure 1.**
*Excess concentration of positive ions, (N+—N−), vs. distance, d. dx is the double layer thickness. The surfaces have different charge density. The difference among them, is dσ. The same holds in case of excess negative charges.*

it is enough adding salt in excess. The potential is screened and repulsion between particles substantially minimized. In this way, colloids do not "feel" each other as it was before adding swamping electrolytes.

The problem can be properly addressed discussing the case of surface charge density, $\sigma$. As a consequence of Eq. (1), $\psi$ decreases with distance. On moving from a reference point, $x^{\circ}$, to $x$, $\sigma$ decreases. The system behaves as a capacitor, and the local, punctual, concentration of ions, $\rho$, decreases with $x$. This is expressed by writing the integral of $\sigma$ from $x^{\circ}$ to the point of interest as

$$\sigma = -\int \rho dx \tag{3}$$

The meaning of Eqs. (2) and (3) is visualized in **Figure 1**. At long, on a molecular scale, distances the value of the integral in Eq. (3) approaches the equilibrium ionic concentration, and electro-neutrality is thus ensured. Therefore, $(N^{+}—N^{-})$ values in the above figure refer to the excess of counter-ions around a given charged body. Swamping electrolytes reduce the effect of potential at long distances and favor coalescence.

In many procedures intended for food chemistry, for instance, salting is by far the preferred route to reduce repulsive forces between entities in the given medium and to induce phase separation [18].

## 3. Sterical stabilization

The role that such effect plays in controlling colloid stability, with particular emphasis to biological systems is considered [19]. The concept was originally intended to latexes stabilization, and later extended to bio-systems. The term "*sterical stabilization*" indicates that macromolecules protect particles from flocculation, or coagulation. It applies to systems in which stabilizers are surface bound to the particles in question, which would flocculate if not protected. Sterical stabilization is intended to systems in which binding to a given surface is permanent. When binding is covalent, the drawbacks inherent to depletion [20, 21], which occurs when the stabilizer is weakly bound and may transfer toward the bulk, are missing. In that case, stabilizers partition between the particle surface and the bulk. This favors the onset of osmotic gradients, detaching stabilizers from the particle' surface with coagulation of no longer stabilized colloids. Predicting sterical stabilization is cumbersome if all these effects are not accounted for. As a matter of fact, polymer moieties protruding outward a given particle are solvated, sometimes charged; their state, conformation and degrees of freedom jointly depend on polymer-medium interactions. In other words, entropic contributions are not only due to changes in conformational degrees of freedom, as proposed by van der Waals's school [22, 23]. More precisely, the Gibbs energy, due to entropic and also enthalpy-based terms [24–26], is the result of different contributions.

We consider the following entropic terms

$$\Delta S_{tot} = \Delta S_{conform} + \Delta S_{solv} + other\ \Delta S\ terms \tag{4}$$

where the subscripts indicate conformational, solvation, and all other contributions, respectively. We do not consider, in a first stage, terms due to charging/discharging of polar moieties. Neither shall we consider osmotic repulsion, which is significant when the "coronas" surrounding the nanoparticles are compact. The requirements needed to have effective repulsion between polymer moieties, and in coronas stabilization too, crucially depend on the solvent. It is not casual, thus, that different stabilizers are needed to disperse colloids in polar, or non-polar, media.

The original hypothesis by van der Waals, which relies only on conformational entropy, is not convincing, since the contribution due to the solvent cannot be null. In fact, the solvent features are responsible for a number of formulation possibilities, including those intended to bio-systems.

To come in more details on the basics of steric stabilization, we report some details describing the first stages of surface anchoring, i.e., polymer wrapping. That process is responsible for macromolecule binding thereon, and not only. We describe below that effect, without entering in much details as to whether binding is covalent or not. Imagine a homo-polymer binding onto a solid surface; in consequence of that, units in the chain face outward, and may bind in a second place. The only physical restriction is that chains cannot enter the particle but may substantially adsorb thereon in many points. The process depends on polymer affinity toward the surface; in words, surface coverage is dictated by thermodynamics. We assume that:

a. polymers and colloidal nano-particles, *NP*s, are mono-disperse;

b. polymer size is << *NP*s radius;

c. wrapping units are much shorter than the fully extended polymer one;

d. different parts of the same polymer may wrap;

e. partition between bulk and surface-bound states may occur.

We impose $X_f$ to be the overall mole fraction of polymer molecules in the medium; it is either free or interacting with particles. The latter is the sum of wrapping and protruding parts. Interacting polymers are divided in two classes, i.e., wrapped, α, and protruding, ε (=1 − α), states. The equilibrium between such states, $K_{\alpha,\varepsilon}$, is defined as

$$K_{\alpha,\varepsilon} = \alpha/\varepsilon = \alpha/(1 - \alpha) \quad (5)$$

As in most classical books on Colloid Chemistry ([27, 28], and references therein), Eq. (5), defines the ratio of wrapped to protruded states, and gives a binding probability, *P*, for adsorbed segments. For an *i*th state, it is defined as

$$P_i = k_i \exp^{-[(\pi+w)al_i/KT]} \exp^{-[\eta/KT]} \quad (6)$$

where $P_i$ refers to a state characterized by a length $l_i$, and width equal to *a*. We assume the latter to be the cross section of the main chain, **Figure 2**. Terms *w* and *π* are energies per unit volume. Their balance depends on the dominance of attractive/repulsive forces acting on the *NP* surface. *η* is a rotational energy, when the pre-exponential $k_i$ is a proper weighing factor. $P_i$ depends on the balance of all energy terms acting in the first layer around particles. The forces acting in the corona depend on the average local polymer concentration, calculated layer by layer. This statement is due to the fact that the content of polymer sub-units in a layer depends on surface curvature, and/or bulkiness, as well [29]. Expectedly, the solvation is not uniform along the protruding polymer chains. Similar cases occur when polymer coverage is close-grained and does not allow surface adsorption of other species. Thus, poly-oxy-ethylene glycols, PEO's, and structurally related polymers (mostly PEO-PPO-PEO block co-polymers) are widely used to avoid protein adsorption and find application if biomedical-intended NPs must not adsorb albumin or lysozyme, otherwise easily nucleating onto the mentioned NPs [30–32]. This common application is in use, others are mentioned below.

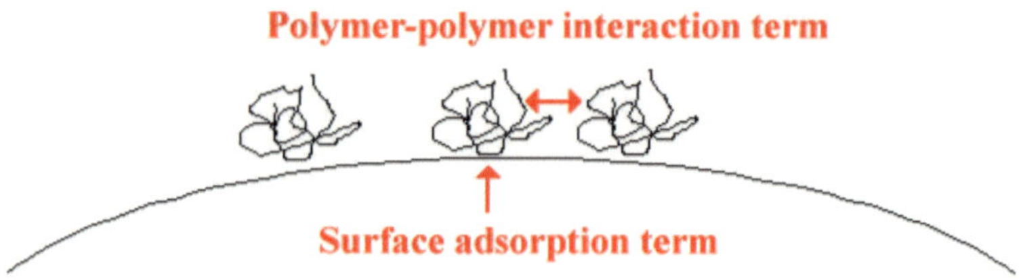


**Figure 2.**
*Polymer adsorption for loops sizes << NP diameter. The surface adsorption term, has energy = w. Polymer-polymer interactions at the NP surface, π, are attractive or repulsive. At saturation wrapping has reached its maximum value. Above that threshold, w and π energies balance.*

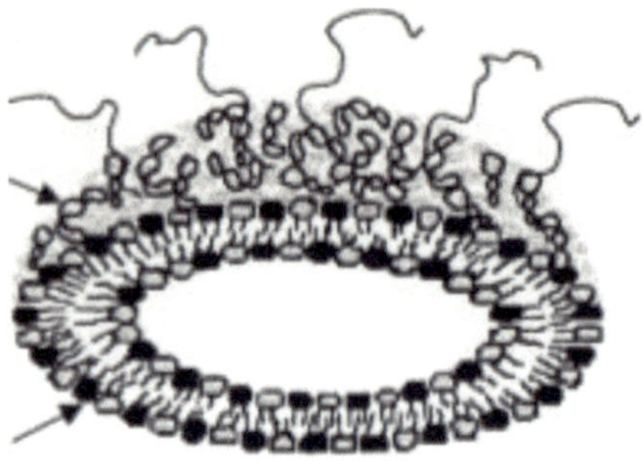

**Figure 3.**
*Reconstructed liposomes with DNA compacted on the outer surface. The lower left arrow indicates lipid head groups; the upper one random coils represents compacted DNA. Protruding whips indicate PEO chains anchored to the bilayer. Such chains are hydrated, elastic, densely packed, and do not allow other species to come in contact with liposomes.*

**Figure 3** describes how to get the stabilization of synthetic liposomes against coalescence and is widely used in transfection technologies.

## 4. Biological implications

Physics and Chemistry allow to clarify some items of biology, despite substantial problems, due to a terrific increase in complexity inherent to living systems. As a matter of fact, these consist of many parts substantially differing from each other, in reciprocal relation. A first glance to a biological sample allows to observe some organization details. Understanding the hierarchy of active forces, packing modes, and processes taking place in bio-systems is discouraging, unless systematic efforts are stricken out. Therefore, most attempts to relate cell complexity to a number of forces acting therein are not trivial. Such attempts require going from simplicity to complexity, and to focus only on the essential modes of interaction. To focus only on the electrostatic and steric effects is a promising starting hypothesis. The first accounts for forces decaying with distance in a predictable way, irrespective of the medium [33]. The second conveys the impression that the geometry dictated by an arrangement of springs, or semi-rigid protrusions, facing outward the particle surface implies repulsion [34]. This fact is more convincing if we account for the additional role of osmotic forces [35], quite often associated to steric stabilization.

Cells always systematically trigger surface charges, acting as a physical barrier against the entry of exogenous material. Passive diffusion is not enough [36], unless it is substantially assisted by other transfer pathways. Imagine having the necessity to insert a nucleic acid in the cell. It is absolutely necessary to make use of chaperons, capable to overcome the protecting action of electric barriers [37]. This action relies on transfection technologies capable to neutralize/invert the charge of hosts to be transferred through membranes, thus favoring uptake. For instance, DNA is neutralized, or adsorbed on oppositely charged vesicles, and transferred into the hosting cells [38–42]. Attraction between cells and transfectants is electrostatic in nature, and its action favors fusion with the cell membrane. It is a phenomenon comparable to the behavior met when viruses enter a cell [43–45]. This mimicry overlaps with other physical effects, due to membrane curvature elasticity [46, 47], its fluid state [48], and so forth [49].

It is known that steric stabilization has a large effect on macrophage uptake in vitro [50]. This effect is tuned by the fixed thickness of aqueous layers, at least in lipid-based chaperones. To ensure long-lasting circulation to immuno-liposomes (and avoid their biodegradation), combination of sterical stabilization with a superior targetability is attained by attaching monoclonal antibodies. These are formed directly on the distal ends of liposome-grafted PEO chains [51, 52]. Similar effects are attained when the more rigid poly-L-lysine is used as sterical stabilizer. In this case, electrostatic effects, due to pH-sensitive charging/discharging of the peptide moieties, are significant. The coupling of antibodies to membranes allow anchorage even in mild basic conditions without the need for antibody derivatization. On the same line, lipo-plexes sterically stabilized with PEO derivatives are used [53]. Relevant are some reports on doxorubicin-loaded liposomes, previously stabilized by adsorption of heparin; these systems show a marked antitumor activity. Heparin is also a coating material stabilizing and protecting liposomes against adverse immune reactions [54], or, in presence of adjuvants, induces drug accumulation at the tumor site [55]. The above list is far from being exhaustive and indicates that steric stabilization, in conjunction with other contributions, is responsible for advanced applications in most fields of bio-medicine and molecular medicine [56–60].

## 5. Final remarks

The "visions" of nature have been different throughout the development of natural sciences. Often physicists, chemists and biologists had a different, sometimes conflicting, way of looking at nature and investigating natural phenomena. One example for all: physical and chemical phenomena (reactions) were considered essentially irreversible in the "classical" history of natural sciences. On the contrary, biological phenomena were considered reversible, and fluidity, change of shape and behavior were dominant. It is not a coincidence that one of the masterpieces of theoretical biology written by J. Monod (1910–1976), one of the most authoritative biologists of last century is entitled "*Chance and necessity*" [61]. As the title suggests, chance seems to rule the biological phenomena: how life arose, the "plasticity" of many biological events. But, necessity is the driving force; a sort of constraint, impeding the same phenomena to escape the stringent laws permitting the completion of a fully functional living organism. Indeed, these strict laws are often represented by physico-chemical (essentially weak) interactions that give a determinant contribution to biological organization and functions. In other words, one could confidently conclude that Occam razor in its popular acceptation, once again, holds true: if there are competing ideas, the simplest one is possibly the correct one. This formulation is not actually the Occam's razor, but rather the law of maximum parsimony. Occam's razor states that in the case of competing hypotheses making the same predictions, the solution with the fewest assumptions is most likely to be true, provided that hypotheses predicting different solutions are not discarded by default. Ockham stated this principle in various ways, but the most popular version, "Entities are not to be multiplied without necessity" (originally "Non sunt multiplicanda entia sine necessitate.") was formulated by the Irish Franciscan philosopher John Punch.

## Author details

Camillo La Mesa[1*] and Gianfranco Risuleo[2]

1 Department of Chemistry, Sapienza Università di Roma, Rome, Italy

2 Department of Biology and Biotechnologies, Sapienza Università di Roma, Rome, Italy

*Address all correspondence to: camillo.lamesa@uniroma1.it

## References

[1] Thompson D'AW. On Growth and Form. Cambridge University Press; 1917

[2] Gros PA, Le Nagard H, Tenaillon O. The evolution of epistasis and its links with genetic robustness, complexity and drift in a phenotypic model of adaptation. Genetics. 2009;**182**:277-293

[3] Rieger R, Michaelis A, Green MM. A Glossary of Genetics and Cytogenetics: Classical and Molecular. New York: Springer-Verlag; 1968. ISBN 9780387076683

[4] Karaiskakis G, Graff KA, Caldwell KD, Giddings C. Sedimentation field-flow fractionation of colloidal particles in river water. International Journal of Environmental Analytical Chemistry. 1982;**12**:1-15

[5] Robins MM. Emulsions—Creaming phenomena. Current Opinion in Colloid & Interface Science. 2000;**5**:265-272

[6] Yasrebi M, Shih WY, Aksay IA. Clustering of binary colloidal suspensions: Experiment. Journal of Colloid and Interface Science. 1991;**142**:357-368

[7] Bell FG. Lime stabilization of clay minerals and soil. Engineering Geology. 1996;**42**:223-237

[8] Luo Q, Campbell DR, Babu SV. Stabilization of alumina slurry for chemical-mechanical polishing of copper. Langmuir. 1996;**12**:3563-3566

[9] Thompson KL, Armes SP, York DW, Burdis JA. Synthesis of sterically-stabilized latexes using well-defined poly(glycerol monomethacrylate) macromonomers. Macromolecules. 2010;**43**:2169-2177

[10] Schill RO, Mali B, Dandekar T, Schnölzer M, Reuter D, Frohme M. Molecular mechanisms of tolerance in tardigrades: New perspectives for preservation and stabilization of biological material. Biotechnology Advances. 2009;**27**:348-352

[11] Crowe JH, Crowe LM, Carpenter JF, Wistrom CA. Stabilization of dry phospholipid bilayers and proteins by sugars. The Biochemical Journal. 1987;**242**:1-10

[12] Kostarelos K, Luckham PF, Tadros TF. Steric stabilization of phospholipid vesicles by block copolymers. Vesicle flocculation and osmotic swelling caused by monovalent and divalent cations. Journal of the Chemical Society, Faraday Transactions. 1998;**94**:2159-2168

[13] Jung M, Hubert DHW, Bomans PHH, Frederik PM, Meuldijk J, van Herk AM, et al. New vesicle-polymer hybrids: The parachute architecture. Langmuir. 1997;**13**:6877-6880

[14] Bloomfield VA. DNA condensation by multivalent cations. Biopolymers. 1997;**44**:269-282

[15] Bloomfield VA. DNA condensation. Current Opinion in Structural Biology. 1996;**6**:334-341

[16] Parsegian VA, Gingell D. On the electrostatic interaction across a salt solution between two bodies bearing unequal charges. Biophysical Journal. 1972;**12**:1192-1204

[17] Fogolari F, Brigo A, Molinari HJ. The Poisson-Boltzmann equation for biomolecular electrostatics: A tool for structural biology. Journal of Molecular Recognition. 2002;**15**:377-392

[18] Vauthier C, Bouchemal K. Methods for the preparation and manufacture of polymeric nanoparticles.

Pharmaceutical Research. 2009;**26**: 1025-1058

[19] Allen TM, Cullis PR. Liposomal drug delivery systems: From concept to clinical applications. Advanced Drug Delivery Reviews. 2013;**65**:36-48

[20] Tardani F, La Mesa C. Attempts to control depletion in the surfactant-assisted stabilization of single-walled carbon nanotubes. Colloids and Surfaces A: Physicochemical and Engineering Aspects. 2014;**443**:123-128

[21] De Gennes PG. Polymer solutions near an interface. Adsorption and depletion layers. Macromolecules. 1981;**14**:1637-1643

[22] Mackor EL. A theoretical approach of the colloid-chemical stability of dispersions in hydrocarbons. Journal of Colloid Science. 1951;**6**:492-495

[23] Mackor EL, van der Waals JH. The statistics of the adsorption of rod-shaped molecules in connection with the stability of certain colloidal dispersions. Journal of Colloid Science. 1952;**7**:535-550

[24] Napper DH. Flocculation studies of sterically stabilized dispersions. Journal of Colloid and Interface Science. 1970;**32**:106-114

[25] Napper DH, Netsehey A. Studies of the steric stabilization of colloidal particles. Journal of Colloid and Interface Science. 1971;**37**:528-535

[26] Evans R, Napper DH. Steric stabilization. Comparison of theories with experiment. Kolloid-Zeitschrift und Zeitschrift für Polymere. 1973;**251**:409-414

[27] Vold RD, Vold MJ. Colloid and Interface Chemistry. Reading, Mass: Addison-Wesley; 1983. pp. 134-148, and references therein

[28] Adamson AW. Physical Chemistry of Surfaces. Vth ed. New York: Wiley; 1990. pp. 421-449, and references therein

[29] Chithrani BD, Ghazani AA, Chan WCW. Determining the size and shape dependence of gold nanoparticle uptake into mammalian cells. Nano Letters. 2006;**6**:4662-4668

[30] Gref R, Luck M, Quellec P, Marchand M, Dellacherie E, Harnish S, et al. Stealth corona-core nanoparticles surface modified by polyethylene glycol (PEG): Influences of the corona (PEG chain length and surface density) and of the core composition on phagocytic uptake and plasma protein adsorption. Colloids and Surfaces B: Biointerfaces. 2000;**18**:301-313

[31] Malmsten M, Linse P, Cosgrove T. Adsorption of PEO-PPO-PEO block copolymers at silica. Macromolecules. 1992;**25**:2474-2481

[32] Docter D, Westmeier D, Markiewicz M, Stolte S, Knauer SK, Stauber RH. The nanoparticle biomolecule corona: Lessons learned—Challenge accepted? Chemical Society Reviews. 2015;**44**:6094-6121

[33] More correctly, the whole process is controlled by the medium permittivity, $\varepsilon$

[34] Liufu S, Xiao H, Li Y. Adsorption of poly(acrylic acid) onto the surface of titanium dioxide and the colloidal stability of aqueous suspensions. Journal of Colloid and Interface Science. 2005;**281**:155-163

[35] Kim S-H, Park J-G, Choi TM, Manoharan VN, Weitz DA. Osmotic-pressure-controlled concentration of colloidal particles in thin-shelled capsules. Nature Communications. 2014;**5**:3068

[36] Di L, PerArtursson P, Avdeef A, Ecker GF, Faller B, Fischer H, et al.

Evidence-based approach to assess passive diffusion and carrier-mediated drug transport. Drug Discovery Today. 2012;**17**:905-912

[37] Valenzano KJ, Benjamin ER, René P, Bouvier M. Pharmacological chaperones: Potential for the treatment of hereditary diseases caused by mutations in G protein-coupled receptors. In: Gilchrist A, editor. CPCR Molecular Pharmacology and Drug Targeting: Shifting Paradigms and New Directions. Wiley; 2010. pp. 460-500

[38] Barbetta A, La Mesa C, Muzi L, Pucci C, Risuleo G, Tardani F. Chapt. VII: Cat-anionic vesicle-based systems as potential carriers in nanotechnologies. In: Ahmed W, Phoenix DA, editors. Nanobiotechnology. UK: One Central Press; 2014. pp. 152-179

[39] Rai R, Alwani S, Badea I. Polymeric nanoparticles in gene therapy: New avenues of design and optimization for delivery applications. Polymers. 2019;**11**:745-780

[40] Shende P, Ture N, Gaud RS, Trotta F. Lipid- and polymer-based plexes as therapeutic carriers for bioactive molecules. International Journal of Pharmaceutics. 2019;**558**:250-260

[41] Bonincontro A, La Mesa C, Proietti C, Risuleo G. A biophysical investigation on the binding and controlled DNA release in a cetyltrimethylammonium bromide-sodium octyl sulfate cat-anionic vesicle system. Biomacromolecules. 2007;**8**:1824-1829

[42] Bonincontro A, Falivene M, La Mesa C, Risuleo G, Ruiz Pena M. Dynamics of DNA adsorption on and release from SDS-DDAB cat-anionic vesicles: A multitechnique study. Langmuir. 2008;**24**:1973-1978

[43] Du X, Wang J, Zhou Q, Zhang L, Wang S, Zhang Z, et al. Advanced physical techniques for gene delivery based on membrane perforation. Drug Delivery. 2018;**25**:1516-1525

[44] Garcia-Guerra A, Dunwell TL, Trigueros S. Nano-scale gene delivery systems. Current technology, obstacles, and future directions. Current Medicinal Chemistry. 2018;**25**:2448-2464

[45] van der Schaar HH, Rust MJ, Chen Chen C, van der Ende-Metselaar H, Wilschut J, Xiaowei ZX, et al. Dissecting the cell entry pathway of dengue virus by single-particle tracking in living cells. PLoS Pathogens. 2008;**4**:e1000244

[46] Temin HM. On the origin of RNA tumor viruses. Annual Review of Genetics. 1974;**8**:155-177

[47] Deuling HJ, Helfrich W. The curvature elasticity of fluid membranes: A catalogue of vesicle shapes. Journal de Physique. 1976;**37**:1335-1345

[48] Winterhalter M, Helfrich W. Effect of surface charge on the curvature elasticity of membranes. The Journal of Physical Chemistry. 1988;**92**:6865-6867

[49] Losa DA, Murata N. Membrane fluidity and its roles in the perception of environmental signals. Biochimica et Biophysica Acta—Biomembranes. 2004;**1666**:142-157

[50] Barbetta A, Pucci C, Tardani F, Andreozzi P, La Mesa C. Size and charge modulation of surfactant-based vesicles. The Journal of Physical Chemistry. B. 2011;**115**:12751-12758

[51] Zeisig R, Shimada K, Hirota S, Arndt D. Effect of sterical stabilization on macrophage uptake in vitro and on thickness of the fixed aqueous layer of liposomes made from alkylphosphocholines. Biochimica et Biophysica Acta. 1996;**1285**:237-245

[52] Bendas G, Krause A, Bakowsky U, Vogel J, Rothe U. Targetability of novel immunoliposomes prepared by a new antibody conjugation technique. International Journal of Pharmaceutics. 1999;**181**:79-93

[53] Sanders NN, De Smedt SC, Cheng SH, Demeester J. Pegylated GL67 lipoplexes retain their gene transfection activity after exposure to components of CF mucus. Gene Therapy. 2002;**9**:363-371

[54] Duehrkop C, Leneweit G, Heyder C, Fromell K, Edwards K, Ekdahl KN, et al. Development and characterization of an innovative heparin coating to stabilize and protect liposomes against adverse immune reactions. Colloids and Surfaces B: Biointerfaces. 2016;**141**:576-583

[55] Park J, Hwang SR, Choi JU, Alam F, Byun Y. Self-assembled nanocomplex of PEGylated protamine and heparin-suramin conjugate for accumulation at the tumor site. International Journal of Pharmaceutics. 2018;**535**:38-46

[56] Merino M, Zalba S, Garrido MJ. Immunoliposomes in clinical oncology: State of the art and future perspectives. Journal of Controlled Release. 2018;**275**:162-176

[57] Rasenack N, Müller BW. Micron-size drug particles: Common and novel micronization techniques. Pharmaceutical Development and Technology. 2004;**9**:1-13

[58] Salem HF, Eid K, Sharaf MA. Formulation and evaluation of silver nanoparticles as antibacterial and antifungal agents with a minimal cytotoxic effect. International Journal of Drug Delivery. 2011;**3**:293-304

[59] Bakowsky H, Richter T, Kneuer C, Hoekstra D, Rothe U, Bendase G, et al. Adhesion characteristics and stability assessment of lectin-modified liposomes for site-specific drug delivery. Biochimica et Biophysica Acta. 2008;**1778**:242-249

[60] Xu X, Ho W, Zhang X, Bertrand N, Farokhzad O. Cancer nanomedicine: From targeted delivery to combination therapy. Trends in Molecular Medicine. 2015;**21**:223-232

[61] Monod J. Chance and Necessity: An Essay on the Natural Philosophy of Modern Biology. New York: Alfred A. Knopf; 1971. ISBN: 0-394-46615-2

Chapter 5

# Self-Microemulsifying System

*Mansi Shah and Anuj G. Agrawal*

## Abstract

Oral route is preferred for drug administration; however according to the recent scenario 40% of new drug candidates have poor water solubility and low bioavailability. One of the biggest challenges in drug delivery science is to improve low oral bioavailability problem which is associated with the hydrophobic drugs due to their unprecedented potential as a drug deliver with the broad range of application. Self-emulsifying systems have been proved as highly useful technological innovations to vanquish such bioavailability problem by virtue of their diminutive globule size, higher solubilization tendency for hydrophobic drugs, robust formulation advantages, and easy to scale up. Self-microemulsifying systems are isotropic mixers of oil, surfactant, drug and co-emulsifier or solubilizer, which spontaneously form transparent micro-emulsions with oil droplets ranging between 100 and 250 nm. Micro emulsified drug can be easily absorbed through the lymphatic pathway and it bypasses the hepatic first-pass effect. Self-microemulsifying system is a thermodynamically stable system and overcomes the drawback of layering of emulsions after sitting for a long period of time. The present literature gives exhaustive information on the formulation design and characterization of self-microemulsifying systems.

**Keywords:** self-micro emulsifying systems, bioavailability, lipid base formulation, surfactant

## 1. Introduction

An advance in in-vitro screening methods such as conjunctional chemistry is leading to publicizing of many potential chemical components with high therapeutic activity. Such rapid identification of highly potent pharmaceutical lead compounds has optimized pharmacodynamic properties but sub-optimal biopharmaceutical characteristics [1]. Most of the drugs are lipophilic in nature and has poor water solubility. Such low water solubility becomes the major challenge in successful development of their oral formulation. Also several drug compounds has low oral bioavailability which further enhances the challenge for the formulator scientist [2, 3]. More than 40% of drugs are lipophilic in nature with poor water solubility. To resolve such challenges, many approaches have been reported to improve the solubility and enhance the oral bioavailability which includes the formation of cyclodextrin complex, lipid based drug delivery system, solid dispersions, micronization, etc. [4, 5]. Among these methods, self-emulsifying systems is one of the most optimistic approaches to enhance the oral bioavailability of poorly water-soluble drugs since it maintains the drug in a solubilized state in the gastrointestinal tract [6]. A stable self-micro emulsifying system consists of mixture of drug, oil, surfactant and co-surfactant. Upon dilution with water it results into fine oil-in-water emulsion with a droplets diameter less than 50 nm [7, 8]. The micro-emulsion droplet of self-micro emulsifying systems entraps the drug molecule completely with 100% efficacy, thus self-micro emulsifying systems shows high potential to deliver low water soluble drug [9]. Rapid emulsion formation helps to keep the drug in a dissolved form and small droplet size offers a considerably larger interfacial surface area which further accelerates the absorption rate of drug with limited solubility. Moreover, the droplets can be rapidly dispersed in blood as well as lymph and the lymphatic drug transport can avoid the first-pass effect [10]. This feature makes self-micro emulsifying systems a significant choice for oral delivery of lipophilic, low bioavailable drugs having ample of lipid solubility [11–14]. Self-emulsifying systems is a broad term which produces emulsions with a droplet size ranging from a few nanometers to several microns. A self-micro emulsifying system indicates the formulations forming transparent micro-emulsions with oil droplets ranging between 100 and 250 nm. Term self-nano emulsifying system is used to characterize the system which results into emulsion with globule size less than 100 nm [15, 16].

## 2. Self-micro emulsifying systems

### 2.1 Classification of lipidic formulations

Lipidic formulations are classified as Type I, II, III, and IV based upon excipients used. Type I formulations are non-self-emulsifying whereas Type II, III, and IV formulations are self-emulsifying. Type of emulsion formed after dilution of self-emulsifying system with water, depends upon the excipients used in formulation. Digestibility of lipidic compositions is also affected by these ingredients. Elements of lipidic systems are represented in the proceeding portion [17, 18]. Classification system of lipid formulation is shown in **Table 1**.

Type I: Drug with tri-, di- or monoglyceride in lipid based compositions is called as type I formulations. Dilution of type I formulations with aqueous media creates

| Formulation | Excipients | Properties | Pros | Cons |
|---|---|---|---|---|
| Type I | Oils lacking of surfactants (e.g. tri-,di- and mono glycerides) | Not dispersing, it needs digestion. | Simple, Compatibility is excellent for capsule. | Formulation has poor solvent capacity unless drug is highly lipophilic. |
| Type II | Oils and water-insoluble surfactants. | SES formed without water-soluble components | Unlikely to lose solvent capacity on dispersion | Turbid o/w dispersion (particlesize0.25–2 mm) |
| Type III | Oils, surfactants and co solvents (both water insoluble and water-soluble excipients) | SES/SMES formed with water-soluble components | clear or almost clear dispersion; drug absorption without digestion | Possible loss of solvent capacity on dispersion; less easily digested |
| Type IV | Water-soluble surfactants and Co solvents(no oils) | Formulation disperses typically to forma micellar solution | Formulation has good solvent capacity for many drugs | Likely loss of solvent capacity On dispersion; might not be digestible |

**Table 1.**
*The Lipid Formulation Classification System: characteristic features, pros and cons of the four essential types of 'lipid' formulations.*

coarse dispersion and is not readily dispersible. Initial digestibility by pancreatic lipase/co-lipase to engender more amphiphilic species is a pivotal necessity for their oral absorption. For potent drugs or drugs with high oil solubility, Type I formulations are preferable.

Type II: These formulation contain drug with oil and water insoluble surfactants (Hydrophilic lipophilic balance <12), and are also called as self-emulsifying systems. Self-emulsification is mainly acquired at the surfactant concentration above 25% w/w. Surfactant greater than 60% w/w that is at higher Concentration, there is formation of liquid crystalline gel phases at the o/w interface because emulsification is impeded. Such systems generate droplets size above 300 nm, when dispersed in water it developed emulsion which is opaque in nature.

Type III: Type III formulations consist of drug, oil, surfactants, and co-solvents for both water-soluble and water insoluble. Ethanol, polyethylene glycol and propylene glycols are selected as co-solvents. Such systems generate droplets size below 300 nm, when dispersed in water and are called as self-micro emulsifying systems. The obtained emulsion is either optically clear or somewhat opalescent dispersion.

Type IV: Type IV formulations consist of drug, water soluble surfactants, and co-solvents. Oil is absent in this type of formulation.

### 2.2 Suitable drug candidate identification for self-emulsifying systems

Drugs that belong to the Class II and Class IV of biopharmaceutical classification system offer potential platform to enhance the oral bioavailability. Log P of the drug indicates the potential utility of lipid based formulation. Maintenance of drug solubility in gastrointestinal tract is the foremost challenges to oral formulation and especially the increased drug solubility at the absorption site of the gut [19]. Lipophilic drug composite that manifest dissolution rate limited absorption, self-emulsifying systems can provide an improvement in absorption in terms of rate and extent, that results in consistent blood time profiles [7, 20]. Problem of poor solubility and low bioavailability of drug across all categories of biopharmaceutical classification system can be resolved by formulating into self-emulsifying system, as shown in **Table 2** [21].

For an oral absorption Lipinski's rule of five has been widely proposed as a qualitative predictive model. In the discovery setting, the 'rule of five' predicts that if there are more than five H– bond donors, it shows poor absorption or poor permeation [22].

Whether solubility and log P are sufficient to identify probable drug candidates for such formulations that question arises and also it is noted that biopharmaceutical classification system and Lipinski's rule of five classification system are useful, particularly at inceptive screening stage, they have some constraint. For recognize the suitable lipid based formulation approach aqueous solubility and log P alone are improbable enough because they do not adequately predict potential in- vivo effects.

| BCS class | Hurdles overcome by SES |
|---|---|
| Class I | Gut wall efflux, Enzymatic degradation. |
| Class II | Solubility and bioavailability. |
| Class III | Enzymatic degradation, bioavailability and gut wall efflux. |
| Class IV | Solubility, bioavailability, Enzymatic degradation, gut wall efflux. |

**Table 2.**
*SES as a solution to various problems to different classes of drugs.*

### 2.3 Choice of self-microemulsifying excipients for formulations

Self-emulsifying formulation produces dispersion in gastrointestinal tract by using different excipients. Isotropic mixtures of oils, surfactants, solvents, and co-solvents/surfactants comprise self-emulsifying formulation and it emulsifies in gastrointestinal tract under a gentle agitation [23].

Depending upon the type of dispersion produced after dilution with water phase, self-emulsifying formulations are further classified as self-emulsifying systems, self-micro emulsifying systems and self-nano emulsifying systems. Emulsion which is slightly hazy, opalescent or opaque colloidal coarse dispersion is called as self-emulsifying systems. Micro-emulsion which is clear or pellucid, slightly hazy, opalescent, non-opaque colloidal dispersion with droplet size below 150 nm are called as self-micro emulsifying systems. Nano-emulsion which clear or pellucid, slightly hazy, opalescent, non-opaque or substantially non-opaque colloidal dispersion with droplet size below 20 nm in diameter called as self-nano emulsifying systems [24]. For the formulation, excipient should be chosen from the list of generally regarded as safe "GRAS" excipients published by USFDA or from other inactive ingredients approved and published by regulatory agencies.

#### *2.3.1 Active pharmaceutical ingredient*

Active Pharmaceutical Ingredient should be soluble in oil phase as this have an impact on the self-micro emulsifying systems to maintain the active pharmaceutical ingredient solubility. Drugs with the low solubility in aqueous media or lipids are strenuous to convey through self-micro emulsifying systems. Exceedingly good solubility in one of the components of self-micro emulsifying systems is require preferably oil phase, if very high dose of drug liked to be administered. For self-micro emulsifying systems, high melting point of drug with log P value around 2 is not appropriate and for self-micro emulsifying systems, lipophilic drugs with the log P values more than 5 are good candidate [19, 25].

#### *2.3.2 Lipids/oils*

In self-emulsifying formulations, oil represents the most important constituent as it solubilizes prominent amounts of the lipophilic drug. Oil promotes self-emulsification and extends the fragment of lipophilic drug transported through the intestinal lymphatic system. Absorption of lipophilic drug from the gastrointestinal tract is enhanced depending upon the molecular nature of the triglyceride used in formulation [26, 27]. Regardless of the noteworthy potential that these lipid excipients have, very few of lipid based formulations has reached to the pharmaceutical market. This may be due to the insufficient data concerning the relatively composite physical chemistry of lipids and scrutinize about formulated drug chemical and physical stability. Incorporation to these studies, its impact on drug absorption is also essential and which depends on interaction of a lipid-based formulation with the gastrointestinal tract environment [28]. Natural edible oils, comprising medium-chain triglycerides, are not commonly preferred in this regard owing to their poor ability to dissolve large amounts of lipophilic drugs [29]. For designing of self-emulsifying systems, varying degrees of saturated and hydrolyzed long and medium chain triglycerides are used. These semi synthetic derivatives form good emulsification systems when used with a large number of solubility enhancing surfactants approved for oral administration. There is polarity deference between the long chain triglyceride and medium-chain triglyceride, a wide micro-emulsion area has been achieved in phase diagram if medium chain triglyceride is used. More is hydrophobic long chain triglyceride, more difficult it becomes to emulsify.

### 2.3.3 Surfactants

The self-emulsifying system demand incorporation of comparatively large amounts of surfactant in addition to the oil, to convey drug in the formulation. Permeability of the intestinal membrane and affinity between lipids and intestinal membrane will be improved due to effect of surfactant. Surfactants improve the permeability by partitioning into the cell membrane and disrupting the structural organization of the lipid bilayer dominates to permeation enhancement [30]. The two major affairs that command the selection of a surfactant enclose first safety and second hydrophilic lipophilic balance. To formulate self-emulsifying systems, Hydrophilic lipophilic balance of surfactant provides important information. High emulsifying performance is achieved if the emulsifier used in formulation of self-emulsifying systems has high hydrophilicity and hydrophilic lipophilic balance. Therefore, for effective absorption at the site, drug is present in solubilized form for a longer period of time and prevents precipitation of drug substance in gastrointestinal tract lumen [31]. Generally single alkyl chains are more penetrative, so surfactants such as polysorbates and triglyceride ethoxylates are found to be less toxic. Usually the surfactant concentration ranges between 30 and 60% of the total formulation in order to form stable self-micro emulsifying systems [32].

### 2.3.4 Co-surfactants/co-solvents

Stress of interface is decrease in the presence of co-surfactant and it allows the interfacial film sufficient flexibility to take up different curvatures required to form self-micro emulsifying systems over a wide range of composition [33]. The mixture with higher surfactant and co-surfactant: oil ratio assists the formation of self-micro emulsifying systems. Disadvantage of alcohol and other volatile co-solvents is that they get evaporated through the shell of soft or hard gelatin capsules and results into precipitation of drug (**Table 3**) [34, 35].

## 2.4 Mechanism of self-emulsifying systems

The mechanism by which self-emulsification occurs is not yet well understood. The entropy change of dispersion is greater than the energy required to increase the surface area of the dispersion at that time self-emulsification is occurring. In a conventional emulsion formulation, a free energy is an energy that required developing a new surface between the two phases i.e. oil and water and it can be narrated by

| Oils | Surfactants | Co-surfactants/ co-solvent |
|---|---|---|
| Cotton seed oil | Polysorbate 20 (Tween 20) | Span 20 |
| Soybean oil | Polysorbate 80 (Tween 80) | Span 80 |
| Corn oil | Polyoxy 35 castor oil (Cremophor RH40) | Capryol 90 |
| Sunflower oil | | Polyethylene glycol |
| Castor oil | D-alpha Tocopheryl polyethylene glycol 1000 succinate (TPGS) | Ethanol |
| Peanut oil | | Lauroglycol |
| Sesame oil | | Isopropyl alcohol |

**Table 3.**
*Example of Oil, Surfactant and Co-surfactant/Co-solvent.*

$$\Delta G = \Sigma N\pi r2\sigma \tag{1}$$

where G is free energy, N is the droplets number, r is globules radius, and σ is the interfacial energy [22, 26]. The oil and water phase of the emulsion separates upon reduction in the interfacial area and free energy of the system. Conventional emulsifying agent stabilizes the emulsion by forming a monolayer around the emulsion droplets and reduces the interfacial energy, thereby provides a barrier to coalescence. For the formulation self-emulsifying systems free energy requires is either very low or positive or negative then, the emulsion process occurs irrepressible. Very low energy requires for emulsification, it involves destabilization through diminution of interfacial regions. It is necessary to not have any resistance to the surface shearing of the interfacial structure to occur the emulsification. Through the emulsification water penetrates into the various liquid crystals or phases. As soon as binary mixture of oil/non-ionic surfactant comes in contact with aqueous phase, formation of interface between the oil and aqueous phases occurs. Aqueous phase penetrates through this interface and starts solubilizing with oil phase till the limit of solubilization is reached at the interface. There is relationship between the emulsification properties of the surfactant and phase inversion behavior of the system.

Upon mild agitation of self-micro emulsifying systems, water penetration occurs quickly and leads to the interference of interface and droplets will be formed as micro-emulsions are thermodynamically stable; equilibrium exists within the system although there is continuous exchange of matter between the different phases [36]. Interchanging of matter usually occurs in two different ways like amalgamation of small droplets followed by the parting of larger droplet into small droplets and fragmentation of droplets which later coagulate with other droplets [37].

Self-emulsifying drug delivery system also poses accountability in contempt of its many assets namely

i. Drug chemical instability

ii. Large amount of surfactant used in formulation causes irritancy in gastrointestinal tract

iii. Precipitation of lipophilic drugs take place when volatile co-solvent is incorporated [38].

## 2.5 Formulation design

Formulation of self-micro emulsifying systems involves the following steps.

1. Screening of excipients.

2. Establishment of pseudoternary phase diagram.

3. Development of self-micro emulsifying systems.

4. Characterization of self-micro emulsifying systems.

### *2.5.1 Screening of excipients*

Selection of the most satisfactory excipients that can be used in the preparation of self-micro emulsifying systems depends on the solubility studies. Solubility of the drug is tested in various oils, surfactants, and co-surfactants [39]. Shake flask method is generally used to performed these type of studies. In these studies excess amount of drug is added to the excipient and then flask is shaken for 48 hours in water bath shaker at room temperature. After 48 hours samples are subjected to centrifugation, then filtered through 0.45 μm filters and drug content is examined [40, 41]. The objective of these solubility studies is to choose oil, surfactant, and co-surfactant that show maximum solubility to the drug. Another objective is accomplishment of optimal drug loading with minimized entire volume of the formulation [42].

To check the emulsification ability, screening of surfactant and co-surfactant is done by mixing known amount of surfactants with equal portion of selected oil and surfactant, and homogenized. The idea about ease of emulsification is obtained when the mixture is added to double distilled water and the number of flask inversions required to form homogenous emulsion is noted [43]. Then, the obtained dilution is tested for turbidity, percentage transmittance and clarity. The surfactant that shows high percentage transmittance at lower flask inversions with high emulsification efficiency is generally selected. Similarly, co-surfactants representing higher emulsification efficiency are selected for self-emulsifying formulation [44].

### *2.5.2 Construction of pseudoternary phase diagram*

Micro-emulsion is formed by the spontaneous emulsification method and can be depicted with the help of phase diagrams. Construction of phase diagram is a useful approach to study the complex series of interactions that can occur when different components are mixed ternary phase diagram is used to study the phase behavior of three components. Ternary phase diagram represents the system with three components oil, water, and surfactant. But in case of self-micro emulsifying systems, the additional component like co-surfactant/co-solvent addition is most common. Ternary diagram contains three corners that correspond to the 100% of the particular component. In case of addition of fourth component, the ternary diagram can be termed as pseudoternary phase diagram [45]. For building of pseudoternary phase diagram, components of micro-emulsion are examined for emulsification efficiency at various compositions. Emulsions, micro-emulsions, micelles, inverted micelle structures may be form and the degree of formation of these structures can be determined with the formation of ternary phase diagram [46, 47]. The fixed ratio is typically formed by the fusion of surfactant and co-surfactant and it may be the mixture of oil and surfactant. This is mixed with the specific volume of the third phase like oil or co-surfactant; then the other component i.e. water is added in a gradual amounts and with every addition the solution is tested for the clarity, dispersibility, time for self-emulsification, and flowability. The total concentration of all components in each mixture is 100%. In pseudoternary phase diagram, the samples which formed clear solution is denoted by suitable symbols in the phase diagram. The area that is formed when these points are joined indicates the mono-physic micro-emulsion existing area and wide area indicates the good emulsification efficiency [48, 49].

The following points may be useful to read and to understand ternary diagram in an easy way. The three corners of the typical ternary diagram represent three components, that is, A, B, and C. The arrow towards BA indicates increase in proportion of A from 0% concentration (at point B) to 100% concentration (at point A), the arrow towards AC indicates the increase in proportion of C from 0% concentration (at point A) to 100% concentration (at point C), and similarly the arrow towards CB indicates the increase in proportion of B from 0% concentration (at point C) to 100% concentration (at point B). It shows in **Figure 1**, composition at point O can be known by the following procedure [50].

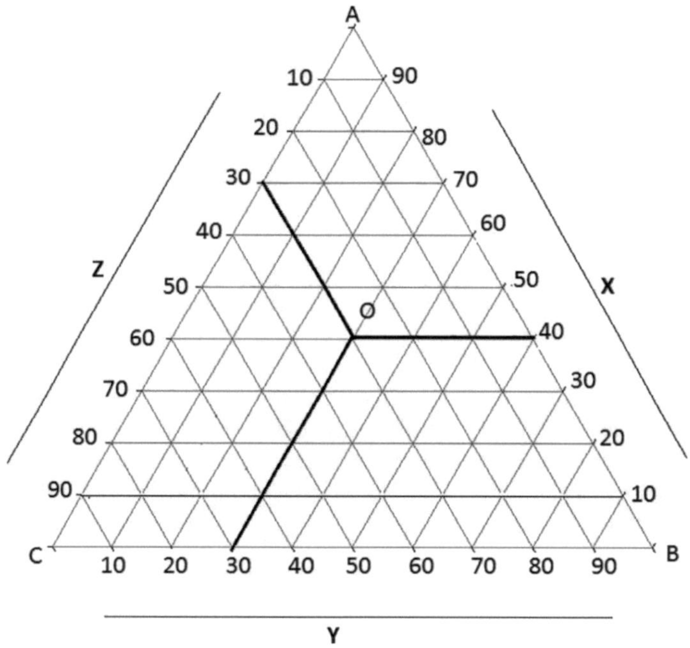


**Figure 1.**
*Typical ternary diagram indicating the composition of A, B, and C at point O.*

i. A line is drawn parallel to CB from point O towards AB. The point where this line intersects with AB indicates the percent composition of A at point O (X).

ii. Then, percent composition of B at point O can be known by drawing a line that is parallel to AC towards BC. The point where this line intersects with BC indicates the percent composition of B at point O (Y).

iii. Similarly, the percent composition of C, at point O can be known by drawing a line that is parallel to AB towards AC (Z).

*2.5.3 Preparation method of self-micro emulsifying systems*

Self-micro emulsifying systems is prepared by adding drug into the mixture of oil, surfactant, and co-surfactant and then vortexed. In some methods, first drug is dissolved in one of the excipients and later on other excipients are added to this prepared solution. Then, the solution is appropriately mixed and turbidity measured. After 48 hours at climatic condition, the solution is heated if required for the development of clear solution [51, 52].

*2.5.4 Characterization of self-micro emulsifying systems*

*2.5.4.1 Visual inspection*

The assessment of self-emulsification is possible by visual evaluation. After dilution of self-micro emulsifying systems with water, the opaque and milky white appearance indicates the formation of macro emulsion whereas the clear, isotropic, transparent solution indicates the formation of micro-emulsion [53, 54]. Precipitation of drug in diluted self-micro emulsifying systems is evaluated by visual inspection. The stable formulation is obtained when drug precipitation is not noticeable. If the formulation contains water soluble co-solvents then precipitation is common outcome and it can be avoided by enhancing the concentration of surfactant [55, 56].

*2.5.4.2 Droplet size*

This is a crucial factor in self-emulsification performance because it determines the rate and extent of drug release, as well as the stability of the emulsion [57]. The droplet size is mainly dependent on the nature and concentration of surfactant. Photon correlation spectroscopy, microscopic techniques or a coulter nanosizer are mainly used for the determination of the emulsion droplet size [58, 59].

*2.5.4.3 Turbidity measurement*

This recognizes efficient self-emulsification by determine the dispersion reaching equilibrium quickly in a consistent time [60]. Orbeco-Helle turbidity meter is most commonly used for turbidity measurements. This turbidity meter is connected to dissolution equipment and emulsification time, optical clarity of nano or micro-emulsion formed is recorded after every 15 second. Turbidity can also be discovered in expression of spectroscopic characterization of optical clarity [61].

*2.5.4.4 Zeta potential measurement*

This is used to identify the charge of the droplets. In conventional self-micro emulsifying systems, the charge on an oil droplet surface is negative because of the presence of free fatty acids. Zeta potential is generally measured by zeta potential analyzer or zeta meter system [11]. Value of zeta potential indicates the stability of emulsion after appropriate dilution. Higher zeta potential indicates the good stability of formulation [62, 63].

*2.5.4.5 Viscosity measurement*

Viscosity of diluted self-micro emulsifying systems formulation is determined by rheometers like brookfield, cone and plate rheometers fitted with cone spindle or rotating spindle brookfield viscometer. During titration, the initial increase in viscosity with subsequent decrease with the increase in water volume attributes to water percolation threshold. This indicates the formation of o/w micro-emulsion from w/o micro-emulsion with intermediate bi-continuous phase [64]. Micro-emulsion can be determined by the graph plotted between shear stress and shear rate. The Newtonian behavior indicates the presence of droplets of small and spherical shape.

*2.5.4.6 Determination of emulsification time*

Efficiency of emulsification of various compositions of medium chain triglyceride systems is determined by using a rotating paddle to assist emulsification in a crude nephelometer [65]. This empowers an assessment of the time taken for emulsification.

*2.5.4.7 Cloud point determination*

Cloud point is generally determined by gradually increasing the temperature of water bath in which the formulation is placed and measured spectrophotometrically.

The point where percentage transmittance decreases signifies the cloud point that is the temperature above which the transparent solution changes to cloudy solution. As the body temperature is 37°C, formulations should exhibit the cloud point more than body temperature to retain its self-emulsification property. Phase separation and decrease in drug solubilization are commonly observed at higher temperature than the cloud point due to the susceptibility of surfactant to dehydration. Cloud point is influenced by drug lipophilicity and other formulation components [66].

*2.5.4.8 Cryo-transmission electron microscopy studies*

Transmission electron microscope is used to characterize the sample. In this sample is taken on copper grid. Filter paper is used to form the thin liquid film on the grid. The grid is extinguished in liquid ethane at −180°C and transferred to liquid nitrogen at −196°C [67, 68].

*2.5.4.9 Percent transmission*

This test gives the indication of transparency of diluted self-micro emulsifying systems formulation. It is determined spectrophotometrically after dilution of formulation with water, keeping water as blank. The percentage transmittance value near to 100% indicates clear and transparent micro-emulsion formation [69].

*2.5.4.10 Small-angle neutron scattering*

Size and shape of the droplets is determined using small angle neutron scattering. Small-angle neutron scattering experiments use the interference effect of wave lets scattered from different materials in a sample with the different scattering length densities.

*2.5.4.11 Thermodynamic stability study*

These studies are useful to evaluate the consequence of temperature change on formulation. Formulation is diluted with aqueous phase and subjected to centrifugation at 15,000 rpm for 15 min or at 3500 rpm for 30 min. The samples in which the phase separation is not observed further subjected to freeze thaw cycles (−20 and 40°C temperature, respectively) and observed visually. The thermodynamically stable formulations does not show any changes in visual description [70, 71].

## 2.6 Factors influencing formulation of self-micro emulsifying systems

*2.6.1 Drug dose*

Drugs with a very high dose are not acceptable for self-micro emulsifying systems unless they exhibit very good solubility in one of the excipients of self-micro emulsifying systems, mostly in a lipophilic phase. The drugs having a little solubility in water and lipids (log P values of approximately 2) are very difficult to deliver by self-micro emulsifying systems.

*2.6.2 Drug solubility*

Solubility of the drug in oil phase is important parameter in self-micro emulsifying systems formulation to maintain the drug solubility. A chance of precipitation is probably higher if contribution of surfactant and co-surfactant is greater in formulation. Dilution of self-micro emulsifying systems will owe to decrease solvent capacity of the surfactant or co-surfactant. An equilibrium solubility measurement is carried out to predict the potential cases of precipitation in the gut region.

#### *2.6.3 Polarity of lipid phase*

Drug release from the self-micro emulsifying systems is mainly affected by the polarity of the lipid phase. The polarity of the droplet is governed by the hydrophilic lipophilic balance, the chain length and degree of unsaturation of the fatty acid, the molecular weight of the hydrophilic portion and the concentration of the emulsifier. Affinity of drug towards solvent is indicated by polarity. Rapid release of the drug in the aqueous phase is high if the polarity is high.

### **2.7 Significance of self-micro emulsifying systems**

1. Self-micro emulsifying systems have the same advantage as emulsions, of facilitating the solubility of hydrophobic drugs. Macro-emulsions undergo creaming over a period of time, whereas self-micro emulsifying systems being thermodynamically stable can be stored easily [22].

2. Most of the self-micro emulsifying systems formulations are in capsule or tablet dosage forms, thus occupying smaller volume, easy to administer and hence improved patient compliance [72].

3. Self-micro emulsifying systems are advantageous over self-emulsifying systems as the former is less dependent on bile salts for the formation of droplets [73].

4. Drugs which have propensity to be degraded by the chemical and enzymatic means in gastrointestinal tract can be protected by the formulation of self-micro emulsifying systems as the drug will be presented to the body in oil droplets [74].

5. Self-micro emulsifying systems have the ability to facilitate rapid oral absorption of the drug, which results in quick onset of action [75].

6. Absorption of drug from self-micro emulsifying systems formulation is not affected by food. The lipophilic contents of fatty diet, aids in absorption of drug from these systems [76].

7. Self-micro emulsifying systems can be easily manufactured at large scale as it requires simple and economical manufacturing facilities, such as simple mixer with an agitator and volumetric liquid filling equipment [77].

8. Surfactants of high hydrophilic lipophilic balance like polysorbate 80 are reported to increase the permeability of the drug when administered along with the formulation due to the loosening effect of these on tight junctions [78].

### **2.8 Challenges in self-micro emulsifying systems formulation**

1. In gastrointestinal tract fluid, diluted self-micro emulsifying systems undergo precipitation of drug. An essential for the lipid formulations is that they should allow keeping the drug in the solubilized form in the gastrointestinal tract. Advantage of lipid-based formulation is abolished due to the precipitation of

the drug. The precipitation tendency of the drug on dilution is higher due to the dilution effect of the hydrophilic solvent. It thereby requires incorporation of polymers to minimize drug precipitation in-vivo [79, 80].

2. Liquid self-micro emulsifying systems are difficult during handling, storage and stability. Therefor formulating solid self-micro emulsifying systems seems to be a logical solution for these problems [81]. Another hurdle in the development of self-micro emulsifying systems and other lipid-based formulations is the lack of good established in-vitro models for the assessment of the formulations [79].

3. Conventional dissolution methods do not work, as these formulations potentially are dependent on digestion of lipid in the gut, earlier to release of the drug. In-vitro model replicating the digestive processes of the duodenum has been developed to mimic the condition [81]. This model also needs more clarification and validation before its strength are examined. Further, development can be based on in vitro–in-vivo correlations.

4. Lipid excipients containing unsaturated fatty acids and its derivatives are prone to lipid oxidation [81]. Inclusion of Lipid soluble antioxidant in formulation of capsule [82]. Polymorphism associated with thermo-softening lipid excipients requires specific process control in their application, in order to minimize polymorphic changes of the excipient matrix.

## 2.9 Patented conventional self-micro emulsifying systems of lipophilic drugs

Self-micro emulsifying systems patent are shown in **Table 4** [83–86].

| Sr. no | Summary of invention | Application | Patent number |
|---|---|---|---|
| 1 | Self-microemulsifying formulation containing taxoid, surfactant, and Co-surfactant [22]. | Poorly water soluble compounds Taxoids having high molecular weight, and slightly lipophilic. This patent enhances oral bioavailability of taxoids through self-emulsification. | EP1498143A1 |
| 2 | The self-micro emulsifying Formulation consisting of poorly soluble or insoluble drug, vitamin E, a co-solvent, bile salt(s), TPGS, and a surfactant [72]. | Increases bioavailability of poorly soluble drugs of paclitaxel and docetaxel. | EP1340497A1 |
| 3 | Self-emulsifying pharmaceutical Composition containing a lipophilic drug, surfactant(s), and hydrophilic carrier(s) [73]. | Improves bioavailability of poorly soluble drugs such as cyclosporine, tacrolimus, ibuprofen, ketoprofen, nifedipine, amlodipine, and simvastatin. | EP2062571A1 |
| 4 | Formulation containing mitotane, propylene glycol monocaprylate, propylene glycol dicaprate, and polyoxyethylene sorbitanmonooleate [74]. | The invention provides the SMES of mitotane, which overcomes the issue of its low solubility and low bioavailability. | EP2435022A2 |

**Table 4.**
*Patented conventional SMES of lipophilic drugs.*

## 3. Conclusion

Self-micro emulsifying systems drug delivery systems are effective approach for increase the bioavailability of poor water soluble drug. Currently, several formulations have been developed to produce modified emulsified formulations as alternatives to conventional self-emulsifying systems, which provide faster and enhanced drug release. Versatility of self-micro emulsifying systems could be proved if issues like method to predict solubilization state of the drug in-vivo, interaction of lipid systems with components of capsule shell and basic mechanism of transport of self-micro emulsifying systems through gastrointestinal tract are adequately addressed. Further research in developing self-micro emulsifying systems with surfactants of low toxicity and to develop in-vitro methods to better understand the in-vivo fate of these formulations can maximize the availability of self-micro emulsifying systems in market.

## Conflict of interest

The authors declare that there is no conflict of interests regarding the publication of this paper.

## Author details

Mansi Shah[1] and Anuj G. Agrawal[2]*

1 Parul Institute of Pharmacy and Research, Parul University, Vadodara, Gujarat, India

2 Netsurf Research Lab Pvt. Ltd., Pune, Maharashtra, India

*Address all correspondence to: royalanuj@yahoo.co.in

## References

[1] Avasarala H, Dinakaran SK, Kakaraparthy R, Jayanti VR. Self-emulsifying drug delivery system for enhanced solubility of asenapine maleate: Design, characterisation, in vitro, ex vivo and in vivo appraisal. Drug Development and Industrial Pharmacy. 2019;**45**(4):548-559. DOI: 10.1080/03639045.2019.1567758

[2] Nardin I, Köllner S. Successful development of oral SEDDS: Screening of excipients from the industrial point of view. Advanced Drug Delivery Reviews. 2018;**18**:30282-30285. DOI: 10.1016/j.addr.2018.10.014

[3] Mahmooda A, Bernkop-Schnurch AM. SEDDS: A game changing approach for the oral administration of hydrophilic macromolecular drugs. Advanced Drug Delivery Reviews. 2019;**142**:91-101. DOI: 10.1016/j.addr.2018.07.001

[4] Karwal R, Garg T, Rath G, Markandeywar TS. Systems (SEDDSS) to enhance the bioavailability of poorly water-soluble drugs. Critical Reviews in Therapeutic Drug Carrier Systems. 2016;**1**:1-39. DOI: 10.1615/CritRevTherDrugCarrierSyst.v33.i1.20

[5] Quan G, Niu B, Singh V, Zhou Y, Wu C, Pan X, et al. Solid self-micro-emulsifying drug delivery system: Precipitation inhibition and bioavailability enhancement. International Journal of Nanomedicine. 2017;**12**:8801-8811. DOI: 10.2147/IJN.S149717

[6] Lan W, Yanli Q, Lina W, Jiahua G, Guocheng W, Lifang Y, et al. A self-micro emulsifying drug delivery system (SMEDDS) for a novel medicative compound against depression: A preparation and bioavailability study in rats. AAPS PharmSciTech. 2015;**16**(5):1051-1058. DOI: 10.1208/s12249-014-0280-y

[7] Phan TNQ, Le-Vinh B, Efiana NA, Bernkop-Schnürch A. Oral self-emulsifying delivery systems for systemic administration of therapeutic proteins: Science fiction? Journal of Drug Targeting. 2019;**27**(9):1017-1024. DOI: 10.1080/1061186x.2019.1584200

[8] Shakeel F, Alam P, Anwer MK, Alanazi SA, Alsarra IA, Alqarni MH. Wound healing evaluation of self-nano emulsifying drug delivery system containing Piper cubeba essential oil. 3 Biotech. 2019;**9**(3):82. DOI: 10.1007/s13205-019-1630-y

[9] Amri A, Le-Clanche S, Therond P, Bonnefont-Rousselot D, Borderie D, Lai-Kuen R. Resveratrol self-emulsifying system increases the uptake by endothelial cells and improves protectionagainst oxidative stress-mediated death. European Journal of Pharmaceutics and Biopharmaceutics. 2014;**86**(3):418-426. DOI: 10.1016/j.ejpb.2013.10.015

[10] Cheng G, Hu R, Ye L. Preparation and in vitro/in vivo evaluation of puerarin solid self-microemulsifying drug delivery system by spherical crystallization technique. AAPS PharmSciTech. 2016;**17**(6):1336-1346. DOI: 10.1208/s12249-015-0469-8

[11] Atef E, Belmonte AA. Formulation and in vitro and in vivo characterization of a phenytoin self-emulsifying drug delivery system (SEDDS). European Journal of Pharmaceutical Sciences. 2008;**35**(4):257-263. DOI: 10.1016/j.ejps.2008.07.004

[12] Qureshi MJ, Chitneni MK, Kian WG. Enhancement of solubility and therapeutic potential of poorly soluble lovastatin by SMEDDS formulation adsorbed on directly compressed spray dried magnesium aluminometasilicate liquid loadable

tablets: A study in diet induced hyperlipidemic rabbits. Asian Journal of Pharmaceutical Sciences. 2015;**10**(1): 40-56. DOI: 10.1016/j.ajps.2014.08.003

[13] Pandey V, Kohli S. SMEDDS of pioglitazone: Formulation, in-vitro evaluation and stability studies. Future Journal of Pharmaceutical Sciences. 2010;**10**(3):53-59. DOI: 10.1016/j.fjps.2017.02.003

[14] Weerapol Y, Limmatvapirat S, Kumpugdee-Vollrath M, Sriamornsak P. Spontaneous emulsification of nifedipine-loaded self-nano emulsifying drug delivery system. AAPS PharmSciTech. 2014;**16**(2):435-443. DOI: 10.1208/s12249-014-0238-0

[15] Rani S, Rana R, Saraogi GK, Kumar V, Gupta U. Self-emulsifying oral lipid drug delivery systems: Advances and challenges. AAPS PharmSciTech. 2019;**20**(3):129. DOI: 10.1208/s12249-019-1335-x

[16] Singh B, Rishi K, Raman deep S, Katare O, Bandopadhyay S. Self-emulsifying drug delivery systems (SEDDS): Formulation development, characterization, and applications. Critical Reviews in Therapeutic Drug Carrier Systems. 2009;**26**(5):427-521. DOI: 10.1615/CritRevTherDrugCarrierSyst.v26.i5.10

[17] Pouton CW, Porter CJH. Formulation of lipid-based delivery systems for oral administration: Materials, methods and strategies. Advanced Drug Delivery Reviews. 2008;**60**(6):625-637. DOI: 10.1016/j.addr.2007.10.010

[18] Chamieh J, Domènech Tarrat A, Doudou C, Jannin V, Demarne F, Cottet H. Peptide release from SEDDS containing hydrophobic ion pair therapeutic peptides measured by Taylor dispersion analysis. International Journal of Pharmaceutics. 2019;**559**: 228-234. DOI: 10.1016/j.ijpharm.2019.01.039

[19] Vithani K, Jannin V, Pouton CW, Boyd BJ. Colloidal aspects of dispersion and digestion of self-dispersing lipid-based formulations for poorly water-soluble drugs. Advanced Drug Delivery Reviews. 2019;**142**:16-34. DOI: 10.1016/j.addr.2019.01.008

[20] O'Driscoll CM, Griffin BT. Biopharmaceutical challenges associated with drugs with low aqueous solubility the potential impact of lipid based formulations. Advanced Drug Delivery Reviews. 2008;**60**:617-624. DOI: 10.1016/j.addr.2007.10.012

[21] Lipinski CA, Lombardo F, Dominy BW, Feeney PJ. Experimental and computational approaches to estimate solubility and permeability in drug discovery and development settings. Advanced Drug Delivery Reviews. 2001;**46**(1–3):3-26. DOI: 10.1016/S0169-409X(00)00129-0

[22] Neslihan GR, Benita S. Self-emulsifying drug delivery systems (SEDDS) for improved oral delivery of lipophilic drugs. Biomedicine & Pharmacotherapy. 2004;**58**(3):173-182. DOI: 10.1016/j.biopha.2004.02.001

[23] Foger FA. Pharmaceutical compositions for oral administration of insulin peptides. EP2523655A2. 2012

[24] Ingle LM, Wankhade V, Udasi T, Tapar K. New approaches for development and characterization of SMEDDS. International Journal of Pharmacy and Pharmaceutical Sciences. 2013;**3**(1):7-14

[25] Nielsen FS, Petersen KB, Müllertz A. Bioavailability of probucol from lipid and surfactant based formulations in minipigs: influence of droplet size and dietary state. European Journal of Pharmaceutics and Biopharmaceutics.

2008;**69**(2):553-562. DOI: 10.1016/j.ejpb.2007.12.020

[26] Gershanik T, Benita S. Self-dispersing lipid formulations for improving oral absorption of lipophilic drugs. European Journal of Pharmaceutics and Biopharmaceutics. 2000;**50**(1):179-188. DOI: 10.1016/S0939-6411(00)00089-8

[27] Hauss DJ. Oral Lipid Based Formulations Enhancing the Bioavailability of Poorly Water Soluble Drugs in Drugs and Pharmaceutical Sciences. 1st ed. Vol. 170. NC USA: Informa Healthcare. 2007. pp. 1-339

[28] Odeberg JM, Kaufmann P, Kroon KG, Höglund P. Lipid drug delivery and rational formulation design for lipophilic drugs with low oral bioavailability, applied to cyclosporine. European Journal of Pharmaceutical Sciences. 2003;**20**:375-382. DOI: 10.1016/j.ejps.2003.08.005

[29] Swenson ES, Milisen WB, Curatolo W. Intestinal permeability enhancement: Efficacy, acute local toxicity, and reversibility. Pharmaceutical Research. 1994;**11**(8): 1132-1142. DOI: 10.1023/A:1018984731584

[30] Shah NH, Carvajal MT, Patel CI, Infeld MH, Malick AW. Self-emulsifying drug delivery systems (SEDDS) with polyglycolyzed glycerides for improving in vitro dissolution and oral absorption of lipophilic drugs. International Journal of Pharmaceutics. 1994;**106**(1):15-23. DOI: 10.1016/0378-5173(94)90271-2

[31] Pouton CW. Self-emulsifying drug delivery systems: Assessment of the efficiency of emulsification. International Journal of Pharmaceutics. 1985;**27**(2–3):335-348. DOI: 10.1016/0378-5173(85)90081-X

[32] Solans C, Izquierdo P, Nolla J, Azemar N, Garcia-Celma MJ. Nano-emulsions. Current Opinion in Colloid & Interface Science. 2005;**10**(3–4): 102-110. DOI: 10.1016/j.cocis.2005.06.004

[33] Mercuri A, Belton PS, Royall PG. Identification and molecular interpretation of the effects of drug incorporation on the self-emulsification process using spectroscopic, micro polarimetric and microscopic measurements. Molecular Pharmacology. 2012;**9**(9):2658-2668. DOI: 10.1155/2013/848043

[34] Singh B, Singh R, Bandyopadhyay S. Optimized nano-emulsifying systems with enhanced bioavailability of carvedilol. Colloids and Surfaces. B, Biointerfaces. 2013;**101**:465-474. DOI: 10.1016/j.colsurfb.2012.07.017

[35] Reiss H. Entropy-induced dispersion of bulk liquids. Journal of Colloid and Interface Science. 1975;**53**(1):61-70. DOI: 10.1016/0021-9797(75)90035-1

[36] Bagwe RP, Kanicky JR, Palla BJ, Patanjali PK, Shah DO. Improved drug delivery using micro-emulsions: Rationale, recent progress, and new horizons. Critical Reviews in Therapeutic Drug Carrier Systems. 2001;**18**(1):77-140

[37] Chakraborty S, Shukla D, Mishra B, Singh S. Lipid – An emerging platform for oral delivery of drugs with poor bioavailability. European Journal of Pharmacology. 2009;**73**(1):1-15. DOI: 10.1016/j.ejpb.2009.06.001

[38] Pouton CW. Lipid formulations for oral administration of drugs: Non-emulsifying, self-emulsifying and "self-microemulsifying" drug delivery systems. European Journal of Pharmaceutical Sciences. 2000;**11**(2): S93-S98. DOI: 10.1016/S0928-0987(00)00167-6

[39] Borhade V, Nair H, Hegde D. Design and evaluation of self-microemulsifying drug delivery system

(SMEDDS) of tacrolimus. AAPS PharmSciTech. 2008;**9**(1):13-21. DOI: 10.1208/s12249-007-9014-8

[40] Wang Y, Sun J, Zhang T, Liu H, He F, He Z. Enhanced oral bioavailability of tacrolimus in rats by self- microemulsifying drug delivery systems. Drug Development and Industrial Pharmacy. 2011;**37**(10): 1225-1230. DOI: 10.3109/03639045.2011.565774

[41] AboulFotouh K, Allam A, El-Badry M, El-Sayed AM. Self-emulsifying drug–delivery systems modulate P-glycoprotein activity: Role of excipients and formulation aspects. Nanomedicine. 2018. DOI: 10.2217/nnm-2017-0354

[42] Basalious EB, Shawky N, Badr-Eldin SM. SNEDDS containing bio enhancers for improvement of dissolution and oral absorption of lacidipine: Development and optimization. International Journal of Pharmaceutics. 2010;**391**(1–2): 203-211. DOI: 10.1016/j.ijpharm.2010.03.008

[43] Lawrence MJ, Rees GD. Micro-emulsion-based media as novel drug delivery systems. Advanced Drug Delivery Reviews. 2000;**45**(1):89-121. DOI: 10.1016/S0169-409X(00)00103-4

[44] Cui SX, Nie SF, Li L, Wang CG, Pan WS, Sun JP. Preparation and evaluation of self-microemulsifying drug delivery system containing vinpocetine. Drug Development and Industrial Pharmacy. 2009;**35**(5): 603-611. DOI: 10.1080/03639040802488089

[45] Narang AS, Delmarre D, Gao D. Stable drug encapsulation in micelles and micro-emulsions. International Journal of Pharmaceutics. 2007;**345** (1–2):9-25. DOI: 10.1016/j.ijpharm.2007.08.057.I

[46] Beg S, Kaur R, Khurana RK, Rana V, Sharma T, Singh B. QbD-based development of cationic self-nanoemulsifying drug delivery systems of paclitaxel with improved biopharmaceutical attributes. AAPS PharmSciTech. 2019;**20**(3):118. DOI: 10.1208/s12249-019-1319-x

[47] Lupo N, Jalil A, Nazir I, Gust R, Bernkop-Schnürch A. In vitro evaluation of intravesical mucoadhesive self-emulsifying drug delivery systems. International Journal of Pharmaceutics. 2019;**564**:180-187. DOI: 10.1016/j.ijpharm.2019.04.035

[48] Eleftheriadis GK, Mantelou P, Karavasili C, Chatzopoulou P, Katsantonis D, Irakli M, et al. Development and characterization of a self-nano emulsifying drug delivery system comprised of rice bran oil for poorly soluble drugs. AAPS PharmSciTech. 2019;**20**(2):78. DOI: 10.1208/s12249-018-1274-y

[49] Elnaggar YSR, El-Massik MA, Abdallah OY. Self-nano emulsifying drug delivery systems of tamoxifen citrate: Design and optimization. International Journal of Pharmaceutics. 2009;**380**(1–2):133-141. DOI: 10.1016/j.ijpharm.2009.07.015

[50] Xu X, Cao M, Ren L, Qian Y, Chen G. Preparation and optimization of rivaroxaban by self-nanoemulsifying drug delivery system (SNEDDS) for enhanced oral bioavailability and no food effect. AAPS PharmSciTech. 2018; **19**:1847-1859

[51] Parveen R, Baboota S, Ali J, Ahuja A, Vasudev S, Ahmad S. Oil based nano carrier for improved oral delivery of silymarin: In vitro-in vivo studies. International Journal of Pharmaceutics. 2011;**413**(1–2):245-253. DOI: 10.1016/j.ijpharm.2011.04.041

[52] Kohli K, Chopra S, Dhar D, Arora S, Khar RK. Self-emulsifying drug delivery systems: An approach to enhance oral bioavailability. Drug Discovery Today. 2010;**15**(21–22):958-965. DOI: 10.1016/j.drudis.2010.08.007

[53] Nazari-Vanani R, Azarpira N, Heli H. Development of self-nanoemulsifying drug delivery systems for oil extracts of *Citrus aurantium* L. blossoms and *Rose damascena* and evaluation of anticancer properties. Journal of Drug Delivery Science and Technology. 2018;**47**:330-336. DOI: 10.1016/j.jddst.2018.08.003

[54] Patel AR, Vavia PR. Preparation and in vivo evaluation of SMEDDS (self-microemulsifying drug delivery system) containing fenofibrate. The AAPS Journal. 2007;**9**(3):E344-E352. DOI: 10.1208/aapsj0903041

[55] Goddeeris C, Cuppo F, Reynaers H, Bouwman WG. Light scattering measurements on micro-emulsions: Estimation of droplet sizes. International Journal of Pharmaceutics. 2006;**312**(1–2):187-195. DOI: 10.1016/j.ijpharm.2006.01.037

[56] Akhtartavan S, Karimi M, Karimian K, Azarpira N, Khatami M, Heli H. Evaluation of a self-nanoemulsifying docetaxel delivery system. Biomedicine & Pharmacotherapy. 2019;**109**:2427-2433. DOI: 10.1016/j.biopha.2018.11.110

[57] Abdulkarim M, Sharma PK, Gumbleton M. Self-emulsifying drug delivery system: Mucus permeation and innovative quantification technologies. Advanced Drug Delivery Reviews. 2019. DOI: 10.1016/j.addr.2019.04.001

[58] Gursoy N, Garrigue JS, Razafindratsita A, Lambert G, Benita S. Excipient effects on in vitro cytotoxicity of a novel paclitaxel self-emulsifying drug delivery system. Journal of Pharmaceutical Sciences. 2003;**92**(12):2411-2418. DOI: 10.1002/jps.10501

[59] Subramanian N, Ray S, Ghosal SK, Bhadra R, Satya P. Formulation design of self-microemulsifying drug delivery systems for improved oral bioavailability of celecoxib. Biological & Pharmaceutical Bulletin. 2004;**27**(12):1993-1999. DOI: 10.1248/bpb.27.1993

[60] Gershanik T, Benita S. Positively charged self-emulsifying oil formulation for improving the oral bioavailability of progestrone. Pharmaceutical Development and Technology. 1996;**1**(2):147-157. DOI: 10.3109/10837459609029889

[61] Usmani A, Mishra A, Arshad M, Jafri A. Development and evaluation of doxorubicin self nanoemulsifying drug delivery system with Nigella Sativa oil against human hepatocellular carcinoma. Artificial Cells, Nanomedicine, and Biotechnology. 2019;**47**(1):933-944. DOI: 10.1080/21691401.2019.1581791

[62] Araújo LM, Thomazine JA, Lopez RF. Development of micro-emulsions to topically deliver 5-aminolevulinic acid in photodynamic therapy. European Journal of Pharmaceutics and Biopharmaceutics. 2010;**75**(1):48-55. DOI: 10.1016/j.ejpb.2010.01.008

[63] Pouton CW. Formulation of self-emulsifying drug delivery system. Advanced Drug Delivery Reviews. 1997;**25**:47-58. DOI: 10.1016/S0169-409X(96)00490-5

[64] Agrawal A, Kumar A, Gide P. Formulation of solid self-nanoemulsifying drug delivery systems using N-methyl pyrrolidone as co-solvent. Drug Development and Industrial Pharmacy. 2015;**41**(4):594-604. DOI: 10.3109/03639045.2014.886695

[65] Agrawal A, Kumar A, Gide P. Self-emulsifying drug delivery system for enhanced solubility and dissolution of glipizide. Colloids and Surfaces B: Biointerfaces. 2014;**126**:553-560. DOI: 10.1016/j.colsurfb.2014.11.022

[66] Singh AK, Chaurasiya A, Awasthi A. Oral bioavailability enhancement of

exemestane from self-microemulsifying drug delivery system (SMEDDS). AAPS PharmSciTech. 2009;**10**(3):906-916. DOI: 10.1208/s12249-009-9281-7

[67] Vasconcelos T, Marques S, Sarmento B. Measuring the emulsification dynamics and stability of self-emulsifying drug delivery systems. European Journal of Pharmaceutics and Biopharmaceutics. 2018;**123**:1-8. DOI: 10.1016/j.ejpb.2017.11.003

[68] Shafiq S, Shakeel F, Talegaonkar S, Ahmad FJ, Khar RK, Ali M. Development and bioavailability assessment of ramipril nano emulsion formulation. European Journal of Pharmaceutics and Biopharmaceutics. 2007;**66**(2):227-243. DOI: 10.1016/j.ejpb.2006.10.014

[69] Khan AW, Kotta S, Ansari SH. Potentials and challenges in self-nano emulsifying drug delivery systems. Expert Opinion on Drug Delivery. 2012; **9**:1305-1317. DOI: 10.1517/17425247.2012.719870

[70] Morozowich W. Development of super saturable self-emulsifying drug delivery system formulations for improving the oral absorption of poorly soluble drugs. Expert Opinion on Drug Delivery. 2006;**3**:97-110. DOI: 10.1517/17425247.3.1.97

[71] Jadhav KR, Shaikh IM, Ambade KW, Kadam VJ. Applications of micro-emulsion based drug delivery system. Current Drug Delivery. 2006; **3**(3):267-273. DOI: 10.2174/156720106777731118

[72] Taha E, Ghorab D, Zaghloul AA. Bioavailability assessment of vitamin a self-nano emulsified drug delivery systems in rats: a comparative study. Medical Principles and Practice. 2007; **16**:355-359. DOI: 10.1159/000104808

[73] Woo JS, Song YK, Hong JY. Reduced food-effect and enhanced bioavailability of a self-microemulsifying formulation of itraconazole in healthy volunteers. European Journal of Pharmaceutical Sciences. 2008;**33**:59-65. DOI: 10.1016/j.ejps.2007.11.001

[74] Sander C, Holm P. Porous magnesium aluminometasilicate tablets as carrier of a cyclosporine self-emulsifying formulation. AAPS PharmSciTech. 2009;**10**:1388-1395. DOI: 10.1208/s12249-009-9340-0

[75] Buyukozturk F, Benneyan JC, Carrier RL. Impact of emulsion-based drug delivery systems on intestinal permeability and drug release kinetics. Journal of Controlled Release. 2010; **142**(1):22-30. DOI: 10.1016/j.jconrel.2009.10.005

[76] Chen ZQ, Liu Y, Zhao JH. Improved oral bioavailability of poorly water-soluble indirubin by a supersaturable self-microemulsifying drug delivery system. International Journal of Nanomedicine. 2012;**7**:1115-1125. DOI: 10.2147/IJN.S28761

[77] Porter CJH, Trevaskis NL, Charman WN. Lipids and lipid based formulations: Optimizing the oral delivery of lipophilic drugs. Nature Reviews. Drug Discovery. 2007;**6**: 231-238. DOI: 10.1038/nrd2197

[78] Tang B, Cheng G, Gu JC, Xu CH. Development of solid self-emulsifying drug delivery system; preparation techniques and dosage forms. Drug Discovery Today. 2008;**13**:606-612. DOI: 10.1016/j.drudis.2008.04.006

[79] Zhang P, Liu Y, Xu J. Preparation and evaluation of self-emulsifying drug delivery system of oridonin. International Journal of Pharmaceutics. 2008;**355**:269-276. DOI: 10.1016/j.ijpharm.2007.12.026

[80] Dahan A, Hoffman A. Rationalizing the selection of oral lipid based drug delivery system by an in vitro lipolysis model for improved oral bioavailability of poorly water soluble drugs. Journal of

Controlled Release. 2008;**129**:1-10. DOI: 10.1016/j.jconrel.2008.03.021

[81] Wasylaschuk WR, Harmon PA, Wagner G. Evaluation of hydro peroxides in common pharmaceutical excipients. Journal of Pharmaceutical Sciences. 2007;**96**:106-116. DOI: 10.1002/jps.20726

[82] Bowtle W. Materials, process, and manufacturing considerations for lipid-based hard- capsule formats. In: Hauss DJ, editor. Oral Lipid Based Formulations Enhancing the Bioavailability of Poorly Water Soluble Drugs. Vol. 170. New York: Informa Healthcare; 2007

[83] Cote S, Gaudel G, Peracchia MT. Self-emulsifying and self-microemulsifying formulations for the oral administration of taxoids. EP1498143A12005

[84] Benita S, Garrigue, JS, Gursoy N, Lambert G, Razafindratsita A, Yang S. Self-emulsifying drug delivery systems for poorly soluble drugs. EP1340497A1. 2003

[85] Hao WH, Hsu CS, Wang JJ. Self-emulsifying pharmaceutical composition with enhanced bioavailability. EP2062571A1. 2012

[86] Battung F, Sansoë L, Hassan E. Self-microemulsifying mitotane composition. EP2435022A2. 2012

Chapter 6

# Cyclodextrin Nanosponges: A Promising Approach for Modulating Drug Delivery

*Sunil Kumar, Pooja Dalal and Rekha Rao*

## Abstract

Nanotechnology showed great promise and impact on administration of therapeutic agents owing to its advantages over contemporary delivery systems. Nanoscale carriers like nanosponges represent a novel category of hyper cross-linked polymer structures with nanosized cavities which can be filled with variety of active moieties (hydrophilic as well as hydrophobic). These nanocarriers can circulate around the body until they found the specific target site and adhere on the surface and release the active moiety in a predictable and controlled manner, resulting in more effective delivery of a given dosage. Nanosponge technology helps to reduce drug associated side effects, improve stability, increase elegance and improve the flexibility of formulations, administered orally, parenterally and topically. Among nanosponges, *cyclodextrin-based nanosponges (CDNS)* are smart versatile carriers studied widely for drug delivery applications. Statistically, it have presented that approximately 40% of active moieties marketed currently and about 90% of active moieties in their preliminary phase confront problems regarding to solubility. In the past decade, the number of studies describing CDNS has dramatically increased. In the present chapter, scientists working in arena of nanotechnology can get an idea of fabrication, characterization and therapeutic utilities of nanosponges.

**Keywords:** drug targeting, solubility enhancement, porosity, nanocarrier, controlled release

## 1. Introduction

The development of new active moiety is very expensive and time consuming. Currently, it is estimated the bringing a new portion of active moiety through discovery, development, clinical trials and regulatory approval will take a decade and cost approximately $120 million. Therefore, an attempt has been made to improve the safety efficacy relationship of established drugs using a variety of methods, such as individualized drug therapy, therapeutic drug monitoring and dose titration. The delivery of active moieties at controlled rate and targeted delivery have attracted the attention of research community and hence, pursued vigorously [1–4]. Further, effective and safe delivery of therapeutic drug molecules has always posed challenge for formulation scientists. For this purpose, numerous nanocarriers have been fabricated and explored. Nanoformulations are highly multifunctional delivery systems possessing a range of applications such as enhanced solubility, stability, specific targeting, on-demand release and degradation within suitable period of time [5].



IntechOpen

Nanoformulations and nanoparticles have already been applied as carriers of active moieties with great success; and they have an even greater potential for many applications, like gene therapy, anti-tumor therapy, radiotherapy and AIDS therapy, in the delivery of virostatics, antibiotics, proteins and vaccines [6]. Among the various novel forms of drug delivery nanovehicle, colloidal systems like nanosponges have emerged as promising and potential carrier for promising drug delivery of tough molecules in the past few decades [5] because other novel carrier systems have their own drawbacks enlisted in **Table 1.**

Nanosponges are a new class of structures based on hyper reticulated polymers that have cavities in the nanorange [7, 8]. Nanosponge technology offers pay load of active moieties and thought to help in reducing side effects, increase elegance, improve formulation flexibility and stability. These are non-mutagenic, non-irritating, non-toxic and non-allergenic. In comparison with other nanostructres, NS are insoluble in organic solvents and water. NS are non-toxic, porous, biodegradable and highly stable (up to 300°C) [9]. These nanostructures are able to transport both hydrophilic and lipophilic moieties and improve the solubilization efficacy of drugs. Nanosponge based drug delivery system is used to improve the performance of drugs administered orally, parenterally, pulmonary and topically [10]. Many active moieties with different pharmacological activities, structures and solubility have been encapsulated in NSs, including camptothecin, paclitaxel, doxorubicin, dexamethasone, 5-fluorouracil, itraconazole, nelfinavir mesylate, progesterone, tamoxifen and resveratrol [11]. Further, we acknowledge some excellent reviews that have been published earlier on nanosponges [8, 12–15]. Some of the well-known nanosponges are titanium based NS, silicon NS and cyclodextrin NS [16]. Nanosponges possess various attractive features [17] like

- Can be employed to mask unpleasant flavors and to turn liquid substances to solids
- Targeted site specific drug delivery.
- Being suitable aqueous solubility, the hydrophobic drugs can be encapsulated in these, after mixing with cross-linker.
- Less harmful side effects (since small amount of the active moiety is in contact with healthy tissue).
- Particle size can be varied by using different proportion of cross-linker to polymer.
- Easy to scale-up.
- Simple method production
- The drug profile can be tailored from fast, medium to slow release as per need.
- Gives predictable release.

Despite of these advantages, nanosponges have some limitations also. Only small molecules can be entrapped which depend on loading capacities [18]. Cyclodextrin nanosponges can be categorized into four successive generations, on the basis their chemical configuration and features (**Table 2**).

| S. No. | Novel drug carrier systems | Limitations | References |
|---|---|---|---|
| 1 | Microspheres | Premature release of active molecules, deficient entrapment of active molecules, Expeditiously taken up by reticular endothelial system (RES) | [19] |
| 2 | Liposphere | Weak loading capacity, limited chemical and physical stability during storage, rapid drug leakage, | [20] |
| 3 | Polymeric Nanoparticle | Challenging large-scale up, polymer toxicity, | [21, 22] |
| 4 | Solid lipid Nanoparticle | Insufficient stability and reproducibility, problematic sterilization, low payload | [23] |
| 5 | Nanolipid Carriers | Sterilization difficulties | [23, 24] |
| 6 | Micelle | Not good for hydrophilic drugs | [25] |
| 7 | Dendrimers | Polymer dependent biocompatibility | [26] |
| 8 | Liposome | Weak load capacity, poor chemical and physical stability on storage, rapid drug leakage, | [20, 27] |
| 9 | Niosome | Less skin penetration | [28] |
| 10 | Transferosome | Chemically unstable, very expensive | [29] |
| 11 | Sphingosome | Low entrapment efficacy, high cost of sphingolipids | [30] |
| 12 | Ethosome | Poor yield | [31] |
| 13 | Phytosomes | Low stability | [32] |

**Table 1.**
*Novel drug carrier systems with their limitations.*

| Generation | Category | Sub category | References |
|---|---|---|---|
| First | Plain nanosponges | Cyclodextrin-based urethane nanosponges ether nanosponges, cyclodextrin-based carbonate nanosponges, ester nanosponges | [33–36] |
| Second | Modified nanosponges | Fluorescent carbonate nanosponges, fluorescent carboxylated nanosponges, electrically charged CD-NSs, hydrophobic NSs | [37, 38] |
| Thirrd | Stimuli nanosponges | pH responsive cross-linked CD based hydrogels, glutathione-responsive NSs, aminocyclodextrin nanosponges | [39–41] |
| Fourth | Molecularly imprinted nanosponges | Molecularly imprinted polymers based CD nanosponges | [42, 43] |

**Table 2.**
*Evolution of cyclodextrin based nanosponges.*

## 2. Architecture of nanosponges

Typically, nanosponges have been constructed from cyclodextrin cross-linked with organic carbonates. Nanosponges mainly comprise of three components- polymer cross linking agent and drug moiety [44].

Nature and type of polymer used can impact the formulation and the performance of NS. The selection of polymer relies on the nature of drug and purpose for which drug is encapsulated. For drug targeting the polymer should possess the capacity to bind with specific ligands. The capacity of the polymer to be cross-linked depends on its active and functional groups to be substituted [44]. Polymers used for architecting the NS are include polyvinyl alcohol (PVA), ethyl cellulose, polymethylmethacrylate, hyper connected polystyrenes, cyclodextrins and their derivatives like methyl beta cyclodextrins, alkyloxycarbonylcyclodextrins [45]. Among these, cyclodextrins (CDs) have been the most popularly employed for fabrication of nanosponges. These cone-shaped truncated cyclic oligosaccharides are comprised of glucopyranose units aligned around the hydrophobic cavity that may lodge guest moieties owing to inclusion complexes formation [46]. The basic physicochemical features of CD have been discovered in the early 1950s and since then they have been applied to improve the pharmaceutical and physicochemical properties, like stability, solubility and bioavailability of active moieties [47]. Conventionally, these nanosponges have been applied for decontamination of water [48]. However, nowadays they have been investigated and employed as nanocarriers for drug delivery in the field of pharmaceuticals.

Cyclodextrin complexes prepared with biocompatible hydrophilic polymers have been reported to enhance the solubility of encapsulated categories in aqueous media. Recently, it has been described that, by reacting cyclodextrins with cross-linkers, a new hyper-crosslinked nanostructured material can be obtained; these are termed as nanosponges [49].

Selection of crosslinker depends on the structure of polymer employed and active moiety to be incorporated [44]. Efficient crosslinkers help to transform molecular nanocavities into three-dimensional nanoporous products. By varying the degree of crosslinking, either hydrophobic or hydrophilic matrix can be formulated and possesses ability to entrap targeted moieties. By taking epichlorohydrin as a crosslinker, hydrophilic nanosponges can be developed, which can modify the amount of active moiety release, increase the absorption of active moiety through biological barriers and act as a potential system for immediate release formulations. Other cross-linking agents, like pyromellitic anhydride, diphenyl carbonate, diisocyanates, diarylcarbonates, glutarldehyde, carbonyldiimidazoles, 2,2-bis(acrylamido) acetic acid and carboxylic acid dianhydrides result in hydrophobic nanosponges [16, 50].

## 3. Engineering of cyclodextrin based nanosponges

Nanosponges are synthesized depending on type of delivery system, polymer and nature of drug and solvents [14]. Various approaches used for formation of nanosponges are (**Table 3**).

### 3.1 Techniques for synthesis of cyclodextrin based nanosponges

Several techniques have been reported for synthesis of nanosponges, however melt method and solvent evaporation techniques have been widely reported in literature for preparation of these porous colloidal nanostructures (**Figure 1**).

An account of various methods that have been proposed is presented below:

#### *3.1.1 Melt method*

In brief way, the cross-linking agent is melted with CD and all components are homogenized and heated at 100°C with stirring magnetically for 5 hrs. Then, above matrix is allowed to cool. Frequent bathing is done to eliminate by-products and unreacted components [47].

DOI: http://dx.doi.org/10.5772/intechopen.90365

| Types of nanosponge | Crosslinkers | Example of crosslinkers | Method | Encapsulated drugs | References |
|---|---|---|---|---|---|
| Cyclodextrin carbonate nanosponges | Carbonyl cross-linkers | Diphenyl carbonate, Carbonyl diimidazole, Dimethyl carbonate | Solvent extraction, Thermal desorption | L-DOPA, erlotinib, quercetin, telmisartan, curcumin, reservertol, tamoxifen, paclitaxel, Itraconazole, Camptothecin, | [43, 51–59] |
| Cyclodextrin carbomate nanosponges | Diisocyanate cross-linkers | Hexamethylene diisocyanate and Toluene diisocyanate | Solvent method | Dextromethorphan, Steroids, Dyes and Naringin | [60–63] |
| Cyclodextrin anhydride nanosponges | Anhydride cross-linkers | Pyromellitic dianhydride, Ethylenediaminetetraacetic acid dianhydride | Solvent method | Ibuprofen, doxorubicin, meloxicam, acetylsalicylic acid and strigolactones | [36, 39, 64–66] |
| Epichlorohydrin cyclodextrin nanosponges | Epichlorohydrin cross linkers | Epichlorohydrin | Solvent method | Creatinine, cilazapril captopril and enalapril | [67, 68] |

**Table 3.**
*Engineering of cyclodextrin based nanosponges.*

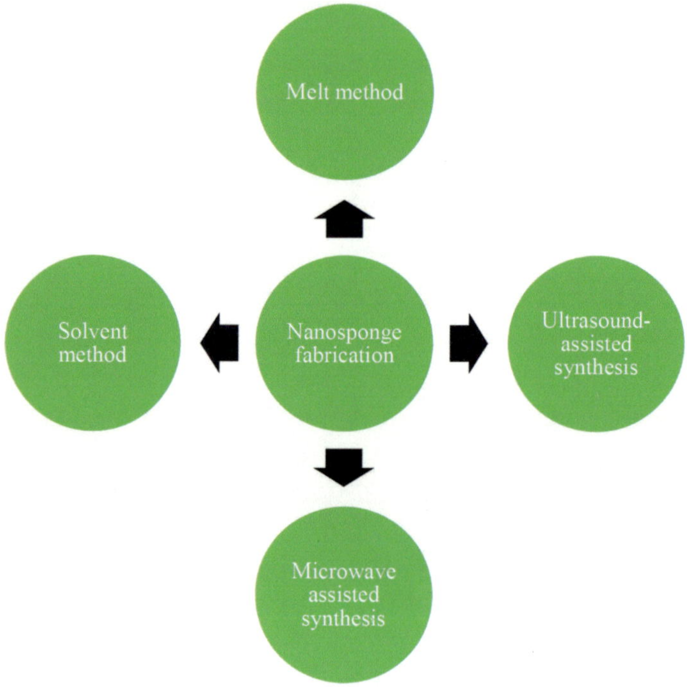


**Figure 1.**
*Various techniques for fabrication of nanosponges.*

### *3.1.2 Solvent evaporation technique*

In solvent evaporation method, the fusion step is avoided and solvents like dimethylsulfoxide (DMSO) or dimethylformamide (DMF) are employed to solubilize the cross-linking agent. Polymer is mixed with solvent (polar aprotic) and the mixture obtained is put in solution of cross-linker and refluxed for 1–48 hrs. By adding cold solution to a large surplus of distilled water, the product is achieved. Finally, filtration is done to recover of the final product and is purified using Soxhlet extraction for prolonged periods. The product achieved is spherical and solid nanostructures with high water solubility either by non-inclusion or inclusion mechanism. The size of NS can be reduced by high pressure homogenization where water suspension of prepared nanosponges is homogenized at constant speed for 10 min [48, 49, 69].

### *3.1.3 Ultrasound-assisted synthesis*

In ultrasound-assisted fabrication, in first, cyclodextrins are reacted with cross-linking agents under ultrasound without solvents. Anhydrous β-CD and DPC are taken in a vial and put in an ultrasound bath, pre-filled with water (at 90°C) and sonicated for 5 hrs. Furthermore, crystallization and purification steps are same as in solvent evaporation and melt technique [70].

### *3.1.4 Microwave assisted synthesis*

It is the simplest method for synthesizing of CDNS using microwave irradiation, remarkably retards the reaction time. The resultant NS possess higher degree of crystallization. In comparison to common melt method, microwave assisted fabrication had exhibited four time reduction in reaction time. The process led to production of particle homogeneous distribution and crystallinity [52].

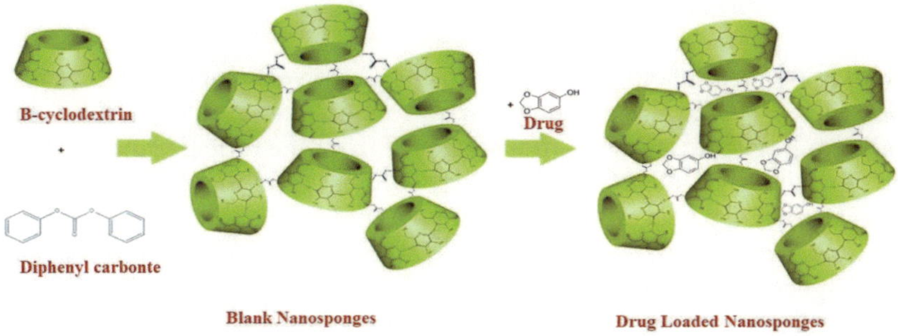


**Figure 2.**
*Schematic representation of engineering of cyclodextrin based nanosponges.*

### 3.2 Drug loading into blank NS

Crystal structure of the active moiety acts as one of the important criteria that determine its complex efficiency with CD and nanosponges. Paracrystalline and crystalline NS vary in the drug loading capacities. When compared, crystalline NS result in higher drug pay load the paracrystalline NS [47, 58, 71]. The porous cross-linked blank NS have numerous interactive sites for inclusion of drug moieties than parent CD. Further, these possess numerous mesh polarities owing to hydrophobic channels of CD which are enclosed by hydrophilic nanocavities of the polymeric matrix, allowing for large interactions with guests of variable lipophilicities and structures [72]. The resultant polymeric network of NS may be responsible for NS protection and solubilization compared to original CD as shown in **Figure 2** [58, 71]. The active moieties are entrapped into nanopores of blank nanosponges by dispersing them within drug dispersion and consequently freeze drying. The solvent evaporation is one another method reported for loading active moieties into NS using organic solvents suitable for dissolving the active moiety. Finally, NS are added to the prepared active moiety dispersion and triturated until the solvent evaporates [47, 73, 74].

## 4. Analytical techniques to characterize nanosponges

### 4.1 Spectroscopic techniques

Spectroscopic analytical tools represent a complementary tool to evaluate nanosponges. The variation in properties such as fluorescence intensity, wave number, absorbance and NMR shift of NS can be investigated by different spectroscopic analytical tools.

#### *4.1.1 Ultraviolet: Visible spectrophotometry*

To analyze NS in solution (liquid medium), UV–Visible spectrophotometry is a fast, simple, valuable and economic tool. The solubilization efficacy of various molecules such as telmisartan (296 nm) [53], acetyl salicyclic acid (234 nm) [65], resveratrol (303 nm) [55], repaglinide (283 nm) [75], quercetin (372 nm) [76] and efavirenz (286 nm) [73] entrapped in NS have been analyzed using this tool.

Anandam and Selvamuthukumar checked payload, stability assay in simulated intestinal fluid, *in vitro* release, metal chelating and photostability investigation for quercetin NS via this spectrophotometeric tool ($\lambda_{max}$ 372 nm) [76].

#### *4.1.2 Fourier-transform infrared spectroscopy*

It is major employed technique for characterization of nanosponges. In general, measurements of FTIR absorption are carried out on dry samples, in the range 400–4000 $cm^{-1}$ [77]. In case of nanosponges, during the reticulation (cross linking), the vibrational modes of cross-linkers, polymers and moieties are displayed from parent positions, broadening or disappearance of the prominent peaks of the molecule, polymer and cross-linkers [78, 79].

In FTIR spectra of the placebo NS, bands that varies from 1700 to 1750 $cm^{-1}$ evidences the carbonate bond. Although, the parent polymer for NS fabrication, β-CD does not show peak at 1750 $cm^{-1}$ in FTIR spectrum [76]. Cavalli and his colleagues explored the occurrence of carbonate bond (1700 $cm^{-1}$) in NS [80].

#### *4.1.3 Raman spectroscopy (RS)*

Nowadays, it is suggested as a useful analytical tool to study drug entrapment in NS [81]. Not only this, it can be employed together with FTIR to provide a better image to investigate interactions of active moiety and NS. Swaminathan and his colleagues performed RS to investigate dexamethasone and nanosponge interaction. On complexation with nanosponges, the prominent bands of the dexamethasone at 1620, 1480, 1440, 950 and 680 $cm^{-1}$ in Raman spectra of the active moiety were substantially masked or displaced, advocating the inclusion phenomenon [82].

#### *4.1.4 Nuclear magnetic resonance*

It is based on the principle of radiofrequency radiation absorption by atomic nuclei having non zero spins in a high magnetic field [83]. Olteanu and co-workers performed the physicochemical characterization of NS using 1H-NMR. High alteration in the chemical shift (0.47–0.24 ppm) of repaglinide A ring protons was observed. It was envisioned that inclusion in hydrophobic pores of CD and steric hinderance owing to CD substitution, have been considered responsible for interaction phenomenon [75].

### 4.2 Differential scanning calorimetry

It is a thermoanalytical technique to measure the change in physical or chemical properties of nanostructures and their fabricating materials owing to alteration in temperature. In general, thermal processes (both exothermic and endothermic) are evidenced by the peak direction [84]. This tool explored the exothermic and endothermic processes at the temperature range from −120 to 600°C [85–88]. The thermal behavior of the various drugs (dexamethasone, furbiprofen, doxorubicin [80], Itraconazole [59], camptothecin [58], resverarol [55], amino salicylic acid [65], gamma-oryzanol [89], telmisartan [53], curcumin [54], acyclovir [37], quercetin [76] and meloxicam [64]) entrapped in the NS was examined by DSC.

The complete disappearance of the therapeutic molecule fusion peak in graph of the NS complex is commonly considered as a confirmatory evidence of the encapsulation of therapeutic molecule within the NS cavity [90]. This may be due to conversion of the crystalline nature to amorphous ones [91]. Other evidence for confirming NS fabrication reported by research scientists include alterations in temperature peak and shape of cyclodextrins, alongwith disappearance of active moiety fusion peak and appearance of new peaks [92].

### 4.3 Thermogravimetric analysis

Thermogravimetric analysis (TGA) is crucial for supply of fundamental data for NS characterization. Due to its very simplicity, relative reliability and rapidity, TGA is widespread approach to solid-state characterization of nanosponges.

TGA chart of dexamethasone, quercetin, silibinin, apple polyphenols NS have been explored. In drug loaded NS thermograms, endotherms of the pure drug disappeared fully, evidencing the potential encapsulation of these molecules in nanostructures [82, 93, 94].

### 4.4 X-ray diffraction techniques

It gives detailed information on phases, texture, structures and other structural parameters (crystallinity, crystal defects and deformation) [95]. Unlikely thermal techniques, sample does not suffer any physical or chemical changes during analysis. Furthermore, XRPD studies can support the results of thermal methods. The complete amorphization of the sample in DSC analysis, can be validated by this technique.

Crystalline and paracrystalline nature of NS and porosity can be revealed using this technique. A number of molecules (acetyl salicylic acid [65], camptothecin [58], telmisartan [53], resveratrol [55], acyclovir [37], quercetin [76], meloxicam [64], curcumin [54], and dexamethasone [82]) encapsulated in nanosponges have been evaluated using this technique.

### 4.5 Microscopic techniques

Microscopy can be used as an imaging analytical technique for qualitative analysis of NS with respect to their aggregation, size and shape. This section provides information on the microscopic methods like AFM, SEM, TEM, and CLSM that are properly used for NS characterization [96].

Scanning electron microscopy is used for observation of surface processes and is capable of obtaining images of bulky samples with a greater depth. It is also employed in solid state evaluation of nanosponges [97]. The topographic changes (related to the interactions of the polymer, active moiety and cross-linking agent) are provided [98]. Various pharmacological active molecules like resveratrol [55], telmisartan [53], dexamethasone [82], and meloxicam [64] have been explored microscopically using SEM.

A nanoscale imaging tool, TEM is used to visualize and characterize various types of nanoparticles [99, 100]. It is relatively expensive and slow technique. Surface morphology via TEM has also been performed for several NS such as ibuprofen [36], quercetin [76], acyclovir [37], paclitaxel [57], dexamethasone [82], camptothecin [58], resveratrol [55], acetyl salicylic acid [65].

Recently developed microscopic technique with high resolution, atomic force microscopy (AFM) is used for viewing atoms and molecules [101]. AFM has been applied to image the molecular nature of β-CDNS in the distilled water and to investigate their mechanical properties. The paracrystalline NS presented spherical colloidal structures (nearly 600 nm), whereas the crystalline NS presented the spectacular crystal planes (nearby 500 nm) [82].

Confocal laser scanning microscopy (CLSM) is recently emerging tool to improve the optical contrast and resolution of sample graph [102]. Lembo and his co-workers examined carboxylated NS loaded with acyclovir for cellular uptake of nanopreparation through CLSM. For this, fluorescent carboxylated NS were prepared [37].

### 4.6 Measurement of zeta potential

The zeta potential (ZP) is employed to measure the electrokinetic potential of nanomedicines. Simply, it is used for quantifying the charge [103]. To investigate the charge on the nanostructures, ZP must be carried out by suspending them in distilled water or suspension medium [104]. CDNS have been evaluated via the electrophoretic light scattering technique [53, 80, 105]. In practice, ZP predicts surface charge and colloidal stability of nanomaterials.

## 5. Nanosponges in drug delivery

Owing to their versatile, biocompatible and nanoporous nature, nanosponges have variety of applications in pharmaceuticals, cosmetics, agriculture, environment, food and polymer industry [55, 80, 106–108]. Among these, they have been predominantly studied for drug delivery. Numerous active molecules including lipophilic and hydrophilic actives and volatile oils can be conventionally entrapped in these multifaceted nanostructures for solubility and stability enhancement and for controlled delivery [7]. Hence, these novel carriers have attracted much interest of formulation scientists as they hold promise in addressing other challenges like poor bioavailability, permeation and therapeutic activity [69]. Cyclodextrin nanosponges have also been explored for drug delivery and drug targeting for cancer management [40, 109, 110]. In the following sections, information regarding their applications in pharmaceutical field has been summarized (**Table 4**).

| Drug candidate | Category | Route of administration | Remarks | References |
|---|---|---|---|---|
| Dexamethasone | Anti-inflammatory | Oral, Parenteral | Improved aqueous solubility | [80, 82] |
| Flurbiprofen | Anti-inflammatory | Oral | Improved aqueous solubility | [80] |
| Doxorubicin | Antineoplastic | Parenteral | Enhanced aqueous solubility | [80] |
| Itraconazole | Antifungal | Oral, Topical | Improved solubilization efficiency | [59] |
| Tamoxifen | Antiestrogen | Oral | Enhanced pharmacokinetic activity of drug | [56] |
| Resveratrol | Antioxidant | Oral, Topical | Enhanced permeation, stability and cytotoxicity against HCPC-1 cells | [55] |
| Paclitaxel | Antineoplastic | Parenteral | *In vitro* enhancement of anticancer activity | [57, 111] |
| Camptothecin | Antineoplastic | Parenteral | Inhibits the adhesion and migration of tumor cells | [58] |
| Curcumin | Anti-cancer | Oral | Higher solubilization potential | [54, 112] |
| Acetylsalicylic acid | Analgesic | Oral | Controlled release | [65] |
| Acyclovir | Antiviral | Oral, topical, parenteral | Enhanced antiviral activity against HSV-1 (clinical isolates) | [37] |

| Drug candidate | Category | Route of administration | Remarks | References |
|---|---|---|---|---|
| Gamma-oryzanol | Antioxidant | Topical | Improved antioxidant potential and photostability | [89] |
| Repaglinide | Hypoglycemic agent | Oral | Solubility enhancement | [75] |
| Apple polyphenols (Rutin, phloridzin and chlorogenic acid) | Antioxidant antiaging and anti-inflammatroy | Topical | High degree of retention and protection | [93] |
| Telmisartan | Antihypertensive | Oral | Improved intrinsic solubility and bioavailability | [53] |
| Efavirenz | Anti HIV | Oral | Bioavailability enhancement | [73] |
| Lansoprazole | Antiulcer | Oral | Prolonged drug release | [113] |
| Tamoxifen and quercetin | Anti-cancer | — | Dual drug delivery | [114] |
| Lysozyme | Antihypcaalcemic | Oral | Inhibit depletion of calcium in antibiotic associated hypocalcemic condition | [105] |
| Meloxicam | Anti-inflammatory and analgesic | Oral | Controlled release | [64] |
| Quercetin | Antioxidant | — | Enhanced photostability and anti-oxidant activity; Improved dissolution profile | [76] |
| Tazarotene | Anti acne | topical | Improved bioavailability and skin retention of drug | [115] |
| Levodopa | Anti Parkinson's disease | Oral | Prolonged release of drug | [43] |
| N,N Diethyl-Meta-Toluamide | Insect Repellent | Topical | Prolong the persistence | [116] |
| Atorvastatin Calcium | Anti-hyperlipidemic | Oral | Bioavailability enhancement | [117] |
| Rosuvastatin | Anti-hyperlipidemic | Oral | Bioavailability enhancement | [118] |
| Strigolactones | Anti-cancer | — | Targeted delivery to prostate cancer cells | [66] |
| *Salvia officinalis* essential oil | Hypoglycemic activity | Oral | Enhancement of stability and hypoglycemic activity | [119] |
| Rilpinavir | Anti-retroviral | Oral | Increased in Bioavailability | [74] |
| Norfloxacin | fluoroquinolone antibiotic | Oral | Enhancement in intestinal permeation and antibacterial activity | [120] |

| Drug candidate | Category | Route of administration | Remarks | References |
|---|---|---|---|---|
| Ellagic acid | Antioxidant, Anticancer | Oral | Enhancement in oral bioavailability | [121] |
| Doxirubicin | Anti-cancer | Oral | Site specific drug delivery | [122] |
| Babchi oil | Anti-psoriatic | Topical | Enhanced photostability, solubility and anti psoriatic efficacy | [123, 124] |
| Imiquimod | Anti-cancer | Toipcal | Enhanced skin retention and permeation | [125] |

**Table 4.**
*Active molecules encapsulated in cyclodextrin based nanosponges.*

## 5.1 Improved stability

Cyclodextrin nanosponges can prevent degradation of drug molecules which are susceptible to degradation when exposed to water, oxygen (air), heat or radiation. Such interactions are being widely studied in nanosponges. The nanosponges safeguard the drug molecules from oxidation, hydrolysis, racemization, polymerization and enzyme hydrolysis [126, 127]. A number of molecules including L-DOPA, resveratrol, camptothecin and γ-oryzanol and have been encapsulated in nanosponges are reported for stability enhancement and reported [43, 55, 58, 89]. Anandam and Selvamuthukumar found that phototability of anti-oxidant drug quercetin increased on incorporating into nanosponges. The main hindrance in its utility is its photodegradation. In addition, dissolution rate of the biomolecule was also remarkably enhanced in quercetin nanosponges.

## 5.2 Enhanced solubility

Poor solubility of BCS (Biopharmaceutical Classification System) class II drugs possesses a challenge in their formulation. However, these drugs can be successfully incorporated into cyclodextrin nanosponges with better efficacy. These nanocarriers improve their aqueous solubility *via* formation of inclusion complexes by enhancing their wetting and solubility in water. The drug dissolution enhancement consequently enhances their bioavailability. Curcumin is a upcoming herbal active drug having potential for treatment of various fatal diseases including cancer. Though, it has higher efficacy and safety profile, its poor solubility and low bioavailability limit its therapeutic application. Darandale and Vavia fabricated cyclodextrin based nanosponges of curcumin to increase solubility and control its release. These nanosponges were obtained using dimethyl carbonate as linking agent. The prepared nanoformulation showed enhanced solubility, prolonged drug release and reduced cytotoxicity against MCF-7 cells. Besides this, other drug moieties which have been successfully encapsulated in cyclodextrin nanosponges for improved dissolution include doxorubicin [80], itraconazole [59], flurbiprofen, dexamethasone [80], telmisartan [53], tamoxifen [56], repaglinide [75] and paclitaxel [111].

## 5.3 Reduction in volatility of essential oil and material handling benefits

Nanosponges have been reported to protect volatile oils against lost by evaporation. These nanosponges can have resulted in long lasting effect due to slow release of chief volatile components of oils [72]. Further, volatile oil liquids (at room temperature) can be difficult to handle and hence needed to be formulate into stable solid formulations. Nanosponges may help to convert these substances into amorphous or microcrystalline powders which are convenient to handle [49].

### 5.4 Modulated drug release

Judicious loading of therapeutic actives into nanosponges ensures a tailored drug release. Developing controlled drug delivery systems is the topic of interest for research community while maintaining therapeutic effectiveness of drug. Employing these nanocarriers ensures optimal drug use with improved patient compliance owing to reduced frequency of administration. Nanosponges showed strong potential for providing sustained drug release in a controlled fashion. Shende et al., prepared meloxicam loaded cyclodextrin nanosponges to enhance solubility and stability and to prolong its release. *In vitro* and *in vivo* results demonstrated controlled release of meloxicam from the nanocarrier for 24 hrs. It was discussed that slow release of drug might have been due to large degree of cross linking that permitted the entrapment of drug as inclusion complex in the nanosponges. Decrease in crystallinity and enhancement in solubility also led to improve *in vitro* release behavior [64].

### 5.5 Drug targeting

Besides enhancing effectiveness of drug, drug targeting also helps in reducing its adverse effects on healthy cells. By using nanosponges for drug delivery, drug is released at the specific site preventing its circulation throughout the body. A limited number of research papers were found on drug targeting using nanosponges. Harth and Diaz have widely explored nanosponges for targeted drug delivery. Polyester nanosponges were fabricated using special chemical "linkers" for delivery of anti-cancer drugs. These linkers ensure that nanosponge bound selectively to tumor cells, on injection. These nanosponges stick to the surface of tumor cells and release the drug in a controlled fashion [128].

### 5.6 Oral drug delivery

Oral drug delivery has been well-established route of administration having high patient compliance. However, delivery of molecules *via* this route poses challenges owing to poor solubility, presystemic activation and inefficient intestinal permeability. Cyclodextrin based nanosponges have emerged as potential carriers for oral delivery without any compromise on safety issues. An excellent mini review on cyclodextrin nanosystems for oral delivery of drugs have been recently published by Adeoye and Cabral-Marques [129].

Zidan et al., have developed atorvastatin calcium for oral drug delivery by encapsulating it in β- cyclodextrin nanosponges cross linked with carbonyldiimidazole. The prepared nanosponges were found to increase bioavailability of drug up to 2.13-folds in comparison to its suspension. In addition, pharmacokinetic studies revealed remarkable decrease in total cholesterol, LDL-C (Low Density Lipoprotein Cholesterol) and triglyceride and improved level of HDL-C (High Density Lipoprotein Cholesterol) leading to improvement of liver steatosis [117].

### 5.7 Topical drug delivery

Nanosponges can also be incorporated in cream and gels for topical delivery of drugs. Although least explored, nanosponges may prove very promising for treatment of skin disorders *via* this route. Besides drug targeting nanosponges also improved drug delivery from topical gel, if entrapped successfully. Nanosponges for topical delivery of drugs have been mentioned for resveratrol, γ-oryzanol, diclofenac sodium and babchi oil in literature [55, 89, 106, 124]. In addition, this nanoformulation also helps to alleviate local irritation problem associated with topical drugs. Conte et al., developed cyclodextrin nanosponges with pyromellitic dianhydride as cross linker and loaded them in semi-solid formulations for skin delivery. Skin permeation studies in diclofenac sodium loaded nanosponge gel and cream gels significantly retarded the drug permeation through skin while enhancing its concentration in viable epidermis and stratum corneum, confirming the localization of highly penetrating drugs in external layers of skin [11].

### 5.8 Pulmonary drug delivery

The pulmonary route is an alternative option to parenteral drug delivery, however, for delivery *via* this route, the drug must be in the form of aerosol. The nanosponges possess the advantage of reduced interparticle attraction forces and better flow characteristics. Further, they possess low bulk density and small narrow dynamic diameter resulting in their greater deposition in lower pulmonary area. For pulmonary delivery, nanosponges of sodium cromoglicate, budesinide, bendroflumethazide using sugar excipients like trehalose and raffinose have been reported [130–133].

Additionally, nanosponges have also been used for protein encapsulation, enzyme immobilization and stabilization. The enzymes like isomerase, hydrolase, oxidoreductase, ligase, and transferase has been studied. Bovine serum albumin when encapsulated as nanosponges resulted in prolonged release [13]. NS can also be employed as carrier of gases like carbondioxide and oxygen. Oxygen loaded NS can be used to supply oxygen to hypoxic tissues in different disorders [134].

## 6. Conclusion

Cyclodextrin nanosponges are colloidal nanoparticles made from inexpensive, biodegradable materials and can be used for internal or external administration. As such, these offer a versatile platform to address challenges like solubility, stability and toxicity for therapeutically effective drugs. Cyclodextrin nanosponges are developing rapidly in the field of nanotechnology possessing several applications in drug targeting, delivery and research, as well as in other fields. Due to their unique porous nature and size-dependent properties, they present the possibility to develop new therapeutic options. Their ability to entrap drugs and controlled release features offer a new mode in drug delivery resulting in higher levels of drug targeting. Therefore, cyclodextrin nanosponges are a great promise to achieve the goal of site specific and controlled delivery aspects and can open new perspectives in the management of complex diseases, in coming future.

## Acknowledgements

The author Mr. Sunil Kumar is thankful to the Indian Council of Medical Research, New Delhi for providing Senior Research Fellowship (Letter No: 45/44/2018-Nan/BMS on dated 14/05/2018).

## Conflict of interest

The authors have no conflict of interest to declare and are responsible for the content and writing of the manuscript.

## Author details

Sunil Kumar, Pooja Dalal and Rekha Rao*
Department of Pharmaceutical Sciences, Guru Jambheshwar University of Science and Technology, Hisar, Haryana, India

*Address all correspondence to: rekhaline@gmail.com

## References

[1] Panchagnula R. Transdermal delivery of drugs. Indian Journal of Pharmacology. 1997;**29**(3):140-156

[2] Rao PR, Diwan PV. Permeability studies of cellulose acetate free films for transdermal use: Influence of plasticizers. Pharmaceutica Acta Helvetiae. 1997;**72**(1):47-51

[3] Rao PR, Diwan PV. Formulation and in vitro evaluation of polymeric films of diltiazem hydrochloride and indomethacin for transdermal administration. Drug Development and Industrial Pharmacy. 1998;**24**(4):327-336

[4] Prasad M, Lambe UP, Brar B, Shah I, Manimegalai J, Ranjan K, et al. Nanotherapeutics: An insight into healthcare and multi-dimensional applications in medical sector of the modern world. Biomedicine and Pharmacotherapy. 2018;**97**:1521-1537

[5] Tiwari G, Tiwari R, Sriwastawa B, Bhati L, Pandey S, Pandey P, et al. Drug delivery systems: An updated review. International Journal of Pharmaceutical Investigation. 2012;**2**(1):2

[6] Singh R, Vyas SP. Topical liposomal system for localized and controlled drug delivery. Journal of Dermatological Science. 1996;**13**(2):107-111

[7] Sherje AP, Dravyakar BR, Kadam D, Jadhav M. Cyclodextrin-based nanosponges: A critical review. Carbohydrate Polymers. 2017;**173**:37-49

[8] Pawar S, Shende P, Trotta F. Diversity of β-cyclodextrin-based nanosponges for transformation of actives. International Journal of Pharmaceutics. 2019;**565**:333-350

[9] Salunkhe A, Kadam S, Magar S, Dangare K. Nanosponges: A modern formulation approach in drug delivery system. World Journal of Pharmacy and Pharmaceutical Sciences. 2018;**7**(2):575-592

[10] Patil TS, Nalawade NA, Kakade VK, Kale SN. Nanosponges: A novel targeted drug delivery for cancer treatment. International Journal for Advance Research and Development. 2017;**2**(4):55-62

[11] Conte C, Caldera F, Catanzano O, D'Angelo I, Ungaro F, Miro A, et al. β-Cyclodextrin nanosponges as multifunctional ingredient in water-containing semisolid formulations for skin delivery. Journal of Pharmaceutical Sciences. 2014;**103**(12):3941-3949

[12] Selvamuthukumar S, Anandam S, Krishnamoorthy K, Rajappan M. Nanosponges: A novel class of drug delivery system-review. Journal of Pharmacy and Pharmaceutical Sciences. 2012;**15**(1):103-111

[13] Jilsha G, Viswanad V. Nanosponges: A novel approach of drug delivery system. International Journal of Pharmaceutical Sciences Review and Research. 2013;**19**(2):119-123

[14] Pushpalatha R, Selvamuthukumar S, Kilimozhi D. Hierarchy analysis of different cross-linkers used for the preparation of cross-linked cyclodextrin as drug nanocarriers. Chemical Engineering Communications. 2018;**205**(6):759-771

[15] Kumar S, Rao R. Analytical tools for cyclodextrin nanosponges in pharmaceutical field: A review. Journal of Inclusion Phenomena and Macrocyclic Chemistry. 2019;**94**(1-2):11-30

[16] Panda S, Vijayalakshmi S, Pattnaik S, Swain RP. Nanosponges: A novel carrier for targeted drug delivery. International Journal of ChemTech Research. 2015;**8**(7):213-224

[17] Yadav GV, Panchory HP. Nanosponges–A boon to the targeted drug delivery system. Journal of Drug Delivery and Therapeutics. 2013;**3**(4):151-155

[18] Vishwakarma A, Nikam P, Mogal R, Talele S. Review on nanosponges: A benefication for novel drug delivery. International Journal PharmTech, Research. 2014;**6**:11-20

[19] Varde NK, Pack DW. Microspheres for controlled release drug delivery. Expert Opinion on Biological Therapy. 2004;**4**(1):35-51

[20] Touitou E, Junginger HE, Weiner ND, Nagai T, Mezei M. Liposomes as carriers for topical and transdermal delivery. Journal of Pharmaceutical Sciences. 1994;**83**(9):1189-1203

[21] Lherm C, Müller RH, Puisieux F, Couvreur P. Alkylcyanoacrylate drug carriers: II. Cytotoxicity of cyanoacrylate nanoparticles with different alkyl chain length. International Journal of Pharmaceutics. 1992;**84**(1):13-22

[22] Cortesi R, Esposito E, Luca G, Nastruzzi C. Production of lipospheres as carriers for bioactive compounds. Biomaterials. 2002;**23**(11):2283-2294

[23] Souto EB, Müller RH. Cosmetic features and applications of lipid nanoparticles (SLN®, NLC®). International Journal of Cosmetic Science. 2008;**30**(3):157-165

[24] Pardeike J, Hommoss A, Müller RH. Lipid nanoparticles (SLN, NLC) in cosmetic and pharmaceutical dermal products. International Journal of Pharmaceutics. 2009;**366**(1-2):170-184

[25] Dhembre GN, Moon RS, Kshirsagar RV. A review on polymeric micellar nanocarriers. International Journal of Pharma and Bio Sciences. 2011;**2**(2):109-116

[26] Barbara K, Maria B. Review dendrimers: Properties and applications. Acta Biochimica Polonica. 2001;**48**(1):199-208

[27] Goyal P, Goyal K, Kumar SV, Singh AJ, Katare OP, Mishra DN. Liposomal drug delivery systems–clinical applications. Acta Pharmaceutica. 2005;**55**(1):1-25

[28] Chandu VP, Arunachalam A, Jeganath S, Yamini K, Tharangini K, Chaitanya G. Niosomes: A novel drug delivery system. International Journal of Novel Trends in Pharmaceutical Sciences. 2012;**2**(1):25-31

[29] Prajapati ST, Patel CG, Patel CN. Transfersomes: A vesicular carrier system for transdermal drug delivery. Asian Journal of Biochemical and Pharmaceutical Research. 2011;**1**(2):507-524

[30] Saraf S, Gupta D, Kaur CD, Saraf S. Sphingosomes a novel approach to vesicular drug delivery. International Journal of Current Research. 2011;**1**(2):63-68

[31] Wahid AA, Ravouru N, Lakshman SR. Ethosomes: A tool for transdermal drug delivery. Circulation. 2011;**3**:14

[32] Suryawanshi JS. Phytosome: An emerging trend in herbal drug treatment. Journal of Medical Genetics and Genomics. 2011;**3**(6):109-114

[33] Li D, Ma M. Nanosponges: From inclusion chemistry to water purifying technology. ChemTech. 1999;**29**(5):31-37

[34] Machín R, Isasi JR, Vélaz I. β-Cyclodextrin hydrogels as potential drug delivery systems. Carbohydrate Polymers. 2012;**87**(3):2024-2030

[35] Rossi B, Caponi S, Castiglione F, Corezzi S, Fontana A, Giarola M, et al. Networking properties of cyclodextrin-based cross-linked polymers probed by inelastic light-scattering experiments.

The Journal of Physical Chemistry B. 2012;**116**(17):5323-5327

[36] Ferro M, Castiglione F, Punta C, Melone L, Panzeri W, Rossi B, et al. Anomalous diffusion of ibuprofen in cyclodextrin nanosponge hydrogels: An HRMAS NMR study. Beilstein Journal of Organic Chemistry. 2014;**10**:2715

[37] Lembo D, Swaminathan S, Donalisio M, Civra A, Pastero L, Aquilano D, et al. Encapsulation of acyclovir in new carboxylated cyclodextrin-based nanosponges improves the agent's antiviral efficacy. International Journal of Pharmaceutics. 2013;**443**(1-2):262-272

[38] Favier IM, Baudelet D, Fourmentin S. VOC trapping by new crosslinked cyclodextrin polymers. Journal of Inclusion Phenomena and Macrocyclic Chemistry. 2011;**69**(3-4):433-437

[39] Trotta F, Caldera F, Dianzani C, Argenziano M, Barrera G, Cavalli R. Cover picture: Glutathione bioresponsive cyclodextrin nanosponges (ChemPlusChem 5/2016). ChemPlusChem. 2016;**81**(5):433

[40] Daga M, Ullio C, Argenziano M, Dianzani C, Cavalli R, Trotta F, et al. GSH-targeted nanosponges increase doxorubicin-induced toxicity "in vitro" and "in vivo" in cancer cells with high antioxidant defenses. Free Radical Biology and Medicine. 2016;**97**:24-37

[41] Russo M, Saladino ML, Martino DC, Meo PL, Noto R. Polyaminocyclodextrin nanosponges: Synthesis, characterization and pH-responsive sequestration abilities. RSC Advances. 2016;**6**(55):49941-49953

[42] Deshmukh K, Tanwar YS, Shende P, Cavalli R. Biomimetic estimation of glucose using non-molecular and molecular imprinted polymer nanosponges. International Journal of Pharmaceutics. 2015;**494**(1):244-248

[43] Trotta F, Caldera F, Cavalli R, Soster M, Riedo C, Biasizzo M, et al. Molecularly imprinted cyclodextrin nanosponges for the controlled delivery of L-DOPA: Perspectives for the treatment of Parkinson's disease. Expert Opinion on Drug Delivery. 2016;**13**(12):1671-1680

[44] Eldose A, Parmar T, Shah H, Patel J, Zala T, Jain H. Nanosponge: A novel nano drug carrier. Journal of Advance Research in Pharmacy and Biological Science. 2015;**1**(7):1-7

[45] Ajinkya K, Prakash K, Vishal P. Scaffold based drug delivery system: A special emphasis on nanosponges. International Journal of Pharmaceuticas and Drug Analysis. 2015;**3**(4):98-104

[46] Caldera F, Tannous M, Cavalli R, Zanetti M, Trotta F. Evolution of cyclodextrin nanosponges. International Journal of Pharmaceutics. 2017;**531**(2):470-479

[47] Tejashri G, Amrita B, Darshana J. Cyclodextrin based nanosponges for pharmaceutical use: A review. Acta Pharmaceutica. 2013;**63**(3):335-358

[48] Trotta F, Tumiatti W, inventors; Sea Marconi Technologies Di W Tumiatti Sas, assignee. Cross-linked polymers based on cyclodextrins for removing polluting agents. United States patent application US 10/510,792; 2005

[49] Trotta F, Cavalli R. Characterization and applications of new hyper-cross-linked cyclodextrins. Composite Interfaces. 2009;**16**(1):39-48

[50] Kaur G, Aggarwal G, Harikumar SL. Nanosponge: New colloidal drug delivery system for topical delivery. Indo Global Journal of Pharmaceutical Sciences. 2015;**5**(1):53-57

[51] Dora CP, Trotta F, Kushwah V, Devasari N, Singh C, Suresh S, et al. Potential of erlotinib cyclodextrin nanosponge complex to enhance solubility, dissolution rate, in vitro cytotoxicity and oral bioavailability. Carbohydrate Polymers. 2016;**137**:339-349

[52] Singireddy A, Subramanian S. Cyclodextrin nanosponges to enhance the dissolution profile of quercetin by inclusion complex formation. Particulate Science and Technology. 2016;**34**(3):341-346

[53] Rao M, Bajaj A, Khole I, Munjapara G, Trotta F. In vitro and in vivo evaluation of β-cyclodextrin-based nanosponges of telmisartan. Journal of Inclusion Phenomena and Macrocyclic Chemistry. 2013;**77**(1-4):135-145

[54] Darandale SS, Vavia PR. Cyclodextrin-based nanosponges of curcumin: Formulation and physicochemical characterization. Journal of Inclusion Phenomena and Macrocyclic Chemistry. 2013;**75**(3-4):315-322

[55] Ansari KA, Vavia PR, Trotta F, Cavalli R. Cyclodextrin-based nanosponges for delivery of resveratrol: In vitro characterisation, stability, cytotoxicity and permeation study. AAPS PharmSciTech. 2011;**12**(1):279-286

[56] Torne S, Darandale S, Vavia P, Trotta F, Cavalli R. Cyclodextrin-based nanosponges: Effective nanocarrier for Tamoxifen delivery. Pharmaceutical Development and Technology. 2013;**18**(3):619-625

[57] Torne SJ, Ansari KA, Vavia PR, Trotta F, Cavalli R. Enhanced oral paclitaxel bioavailability after administration of paclitaxel-loaded nanosponges. Drug Delivery. 2010;**17**(6):419-425

[58] Swaminathan S, Pastero L, Serpe L, Trotta F, Vavia P, Aquilano D, et al. Cyclodextrin-based nanosponges encapsulating camptothecin: Physicochemical characterization, stability and cytotoxicity. European Journal of Pharmaceutics and Biopharmaceutics. 2010;**74**(2):193-201

[59] Swaminathan S, Vavia PR, Trotta F, Torne S. Formulation of betacyclodextrin based nanosponges of itraconazole. Journal of Inclusion Phenomena and Macrocyclic Chemistry. 2007;**57**(1-4):89-94

[60] Hishiya T, Shibata M, Kakazu M, Asanuma H, Komiyama M. Molecularly imprinted cyclodextrins as selective receptors for steroids. Macromolecules. 1999;**32**(7):2265-2269

[61] Roche PJ, Ng SM, Narayanaswamy R, Goddard N, Page KM. Multiple surface plasmon resonance quantification of dextromethorphan using a molecularly imprinted β-cyclodextrin polymer: A potential probe for drug–drug interactions. Sensors and Actuators, B: Chemical. 2009;**139**(1):22-29

[62] Ma X, Chen Z, Chen R, Zheng X, Chen X, Lan R. Imprinted β-cyclodextrin polymers using naringin as template. Polymer International. 2011;**60**(10):1455-1460

[63] Kyzas GZ, Lazaridis NK, Bikiaris DN. Optimization of chitosan and β-cyclodextrin molecularly imprinted polymer synthesis for dye adsorption. Carbohydrate Polymers. 2013;**91**(1):198-208

[64] Shende PK, Gaud RS, Bakal R, Patil D. Effect of inclusion complexation of meloxicam with β-cyclodextrin-and β-cyclodextrin-based nanosponges on solubility, in vitro release and stability studies. Colloids and Surfaces B: Biointerfaces. 2015;**136**:105-110

[65] Shende PK, Trotta F, Gaud RS, Deshmukh K, Cavalli R, Biasizzo M. Influence of different techniques on formulation and comparative characterization of inclusion complexes of ASA with β-cyclodextrin and inclusion complexes of ASA with PMDA cross-linked β-cyclodextrin nanosponges. Journal of Inclusion Phenomena and Macrocyclic Chemistry. 2012;**74**(1-4):447-454

[66] Argenziano M, Lombardi C, Ferrara B, Trotta F, Caldera F, Blangetti M, et al. Glutathione/pH-responsive nanosponges enhance strigolactone delivery to prostate cancer cells. Oncotarget. 2018;**9**(88):35813-35829

[67] Tsai HA, Syu MJ. Synthesis of creatinine-imprinted poly (β-cyclodextrin) for the specific binding of creatinine. Biomaterials. 2005;**26**(15):2759-2766

[68] Olteanu AA, Arama CC, Bleotu C, Lupuleasa D, Monciu CM. Investigation of cyclodextrin based nanosponges complexes with angiotensin I converting enzyme inhibitors (Enalapril, captopril, cilazapril). Farmácia. 2015;**63**:492-503

[69] ChilajwarSV, PednekarPP, JadhavKR, Gupta GJ, Kadam VJ. Cyclodextrin-based nanosponges: A propitious platform for enhancing drug delivery. Expert Opinion on Drug Delivery. 2014;**11**(1):111-120

[70] Trotta F, Cavalli R, Tumiatti W, Zerbinati O, Roggero C, Vallero R, inventors; Sea Marconi Technologies Di W Tumiatti Sas, assignee. Ultrasound-assisted synthesis of cyclodextrin-based nanosponges. United States patent application US 11/630,403; 2008

[71] Cavalli R, Akhter AK, Bisazza A, Giustetto P, Trotta F, Vavia P. Nanosponge formulations as oxygen delivery systems. International Journal of Pharmaceutics. 2010;**402**(1-2):254-257

[72] Trotta F, Zanetti M, Cavalli R. Cyclodextrin-based nanosponges as drug carriers. Beilstein Journal of Organic Chemistry. 2012;**8**:2091

[73] Rao MR, Shirsath C. Enhancement of bioavailability of non-nucleoside reverse transciptase inhibitor using nanosponges. AAPS PharmSciTech. 2017;**18**(5):1728-1738

[74] Rao MR, Chaudhari J, Trotta F, Caldera F. Investigation of cyclodextrin-based nanosponges for solubility and bioavailability enhancement of rilpivirine. AAPS PharmSciTech. 2018;**19**(5):2358-2369

[75] Olteanu AA, Aramă CC, Radu C, Mihăescu C, Monciu CM. Effect of β-cyclodextrins based nanosponges on the solubility of lipophilic pharmacological active substances (repaglinide). Journal of Inclusion Phenomena and Macrocyclic Chemistry. 2014;**80**(1-2):17-24

[76] Anandam S, Selvamuthukumar S. Fabrication of cyclodextrin nanosponges for quercetin delivery: Physicochemical characterization, photostability, and antioxidant effects. Journal of Materials Science. 2014;**49**(23):8140-8153

[77] Ahmed RZ, Patil G, Zaheer Z. Nanosponges–A completely new nano-horizon: Pharmaceutical applications and recent advances. Drug Development and Industrial Pharmacy. 2013;**39**(9):1263-1272

[78] Bragagni M, Maestrelli F, Mura P. Physical chemical characterization of binary systems of prilocaine hydrochloride with triacetyl-β-cyclodextrin. Journal of Inclusion Phenomena and Macrocyclic Chemistry. 2010;**68**(3-4):437-445

[79] Menezes PP, Serafini MR, Santana BV, Nunes RS, Quintans LJ Jr, Silva GF, et al. Solid-state β-cyclodextrin

complexes containing geraniol. Thermochimica Acta. 2012;**548**:45-50

[80] Cavalli R, Trotta F, Tumiatti W. Cyclodextrin-based nanosponges for drug delivery. Journal of Inclusion Phenomena and Macrocyclic Chemistry. 2006;**56**(1-2):209-213

[81] Crupi V, Fontana A, Majolino D, Mele A, Melone L, Punta C, et al. Hydrogen-bond dynamics of water confined in cyclodextrin nanosponges hydrogel. Journal of Inclusion Phenomena and Macrocyclic Chemistry. 2014;**80**(1-2):69-75

[82] Swaminathan S, Vavia PR, Trotta F, Cavalli R, Tumbiolo S, Bertinetti L, et al. Structural evidence of differential forms of nanosponges of beta-cyclodextrin and its effect on solubilization of a model drug. Journal of Inclusion Phenomena and Macrocyclic Chemistry. 2013;**76**(1-2):201-211

[83] Ibañez E, Cifuentes A. New analytical techniques in food science. Critical Reviews in Food Science and Nutrition. 2001;**41**(6):413-450

[84] Biliaderis CG. Differential scanning calorimetry in food research—A review. Food Chemistry. 1983;**10**(4):239-265

[85] Chartoff RP. Thermoplastic Polymers in Thermal Characterization of Polymeric Materials. Academic Press: New York; 1997. p. 513

[86] Bair HE. Thermal analysis of additives in polymers. In: Turi A, editor. Thermal Characterization of Polymeric Materials. 1st ed. Cambridge, Massachusetts, USA: Academic Press, Elsevier; 1981. pp. 845-906

[87] Gallagher PK. Thermal Characterization of Polymeric Materials. San Diego: Academic Press; 1997

[88] Wunderlich B. Basics of thermal analysis. In: Wunderlich B, editor. Thermal Analysis of Polymeric Materials. Berlin, Heidelberg: Springer; 2005. pp. 71-188

[89] Sapino S, Carlotti ME, Cavalli R, Ugazio E, Berlier G, Gastaldi L, et al. Photochemical and antioxidant properties of gamma-oryzanol in beta-cyclodextrin-based nanosponges. Journal of Inclusion Phenomena and Macrocyclic Chemistry. 2013;**75**(1-2):69-76

[90] Chen W, Yang LJ, Ma SX, Yang XD, Fan BM, Lin J. Crassicauline A/β-cyclodextrin host–guest system: Preparation, characterization, inclusion mode, solubilization and stability. Carbohydrate Polymers. 2011;**84**(4):1321-1328

[91] Bettinetti G, Mura P, Faucci MT, Sorrenti M, Setti M. Interaction of naproxen with noncrystalline acetyl β-and acetyl γ-cyclodextrins in the solid and liquid state. European Journal of Pharmaceutical Sciences. 2002;**15**(1):21-29

[92] Wang DW, Ouyang CB, Liu Q, Yuan HL, Liu XH. Inclusion of quinestrol and 2, 6-di-O-methyl-β-cyclodextrin: Preparation, characterization, and inclusion mode. Carbohydrate Polymers. 2013;**93**(2):753-760

[93] Ramírez-Ambrosi M, Caldera F, Trotta F, Berrueta LÁ, Gallo B. Encapsulation of apple polyphenols in β-CD nanosponges. Journal of Inclusion Phenomena and Macrocyclic Chemistry. 2014;**80**(1-2):85-92

[94] Massaro M, Cinà V, Labbozzetta M, Lazzara G, Meo PL, Poma P, et al. Chemical and pharmaceutical evaluation of the relationship between triazole linkers and pore size on cyclodextrin–calixarene nanosponges used as carriers for natural drugs. RSC Advances. 2016;**6**(56):50858-50866

[95] Bunaciu AA, UdriŞTioiu EG, Aboul-Enein HY. X-ray diffraction: Instrumentation and applications. Critical Reviews in Analytical Chemistry. 2015;**45**(4):289-299

[96] Luykx DM, Peters RJ, van Ruth SM, Bouwmeester H. A review of analytical methods for the identification and characterization of nano delivery systems in food. Journal of Agricultural and Food Chemistry. 2008;**56**(18):8231-8247

[97] Fraunhofer W, Winter G. The use of asymmetrical flow field-flow fractionation in pharmaceutics and biopharmaceutics. European Journal of Pharmaceutics and Biopharmaceutics. 2004;**58**(2):369-383

[98] Maestrelli F, Cecchi M, Cirri M, Capasso G, Mennini N, Mura P. Comparative study of oxaprozin complexation with natural and chemically-modified cyclodextrins in solution and in the solid state. Journal of Inclusion Phenomena and Macrocyclic Chemistry. 2009;**63**(1-2):17-25

[99] Williams DB, Carter CB. The transmission electron microscope. In: Transmission Electron Microscopy. Boston, MA: Springer; 1996. pp. 3-17

[100] Wang ZL. Transmission electron microscopy of shape-controlled nanocrystals and their assemblies. The Journal of Physical Chemistry B. 2000;**104**:1153-1175

[101] Ruozi B, Tosi G, Forni F, Fresta M, Vandelli MA. Atomic force microscopy and photon correlation spectroscopy: Two techniques for rapid characterization of liposomes. European Journal of Pharmaceutical Sciences. 2005;**25**(1):81-89

[102] Jonkman J, Brown CM. Any way you slice it—A comparison of confocal microscopy techniques. Journal of Biomolecular Techniques: JBT. 2015;**26**(2):54

[103] Kutscher HL, Chao P, Deshmukh M, Rajan SS, Singh Y, Hu P, et al. Enhanced passive pulmonary targeting and retention of PEGylated rigid microparticles in rats. International Journal of Pharmaceutics. 2010;**402**(1-2):64-71

[104] Radomska-Soukharev A. Stability of lipid excipients in solid lipid nanoparticles. Advanced Drug Delivery Reviews. 2007;**59**(6):411-418

[105] Deshmukh K, Tanwar YS, Sharma S, Shende P, Cavalli R. Functionalized nanosponges for controlled antibacterial and antihypocalcemic actions. Biomedicine and Pharmacotherapy. 2016;**84**:485-494

[106] Montazer M, Mehr EB. Na-diclofenac β-cyclodextrin inclusion complex on cotton wound dressing. The Journal of The Textile Institute. 2010;**101**(5):373-379

[107] Seglie L, Martina K, Devecchi M, Roggero C, Trotta F, Scariot V. The effects of 1-MCP in cyclodextrin-based nanosponges to improve the vase life of Dianthus caryophyllus cut flowers. Postharvest Biology and Technology. 2011;**59**(2):200-205

[108] Seglie L, Spadaro D, Trotta F, Devecchi M, Gullino ML, Scariot V. Use of 1-methylcylopropene in cyclodextrin-based nanosponges to control grey mould caused by Botrytis cinerea on Dianthus caryophyllus cut flowers. Postharvest Biology and Technology. 2012;**64**(1):55-57

[109] Minelli R, Cavalli R, Ellis L, Pettazzoni P, Trotta F, Ciamporcero E, et al. Nanosponge-encapsulated camptothecin exerts anti-tumor activity in human prostate cancer cells. European Journal of Pharmaceutical Sciences. 2012;**47**(4):686-694

[110] Swaminathan S, Cavalli R, Trotta F. Cyclodextrin-based nanosponges:

A versatile platform for cancer nanotherapeutics development. Wiley Interdisciplinary Reviews. Nanomedicine and Nanobiotechnology. 2016;**8**(4):579-601

[111] Mognetti B, Barberis A, Marino S, Berta G, De Francia S, Trotta F, et al. In vitro enhancement of anticancer activity of paclitaxel by a Cremophor free cyclodextrin-based nanosponge formulation. Journal of Inclusion Phenomena and Macrocyclic Chemistry. 2012;**74**(1-4):201-210

[112] Pushpalatha R, Selvamuthukumar S, Kilimozhi D. Cross-linked, cyclodextrin-based nanosponges for curcumin delivery-physicochemical characterization, drug release, stability and cytotoxicity. Journal of Drug Delivery Science and Technology. 2018;**45**:45-53

[113] Penjuri SC, Ravouru N, Damineni S, Bns S, Formulation PSR. Evaluation of lansoprazole loaded nanosponges. Turkish Journal of Pharmaceutical Sciences. 2016;**13**(3):304-310

[114] Lockhart JN, Stevens DM, Beezer DB, Kravitz A, Harth E. Dual drug delivery of tamoxifen and quercetin: Regulated metabolism for anticancer treatment with nanosponges. Journal of Controlled Release. 2015;**220**:751-757

[115] Aggarwal G, Nagpal M, Kaur G. Development and comparison of nanosponge and niosome based gel for the topical delivery of tazarotene. Pharmaceutical nanotechnology. 2016;**4**(3):213-228

[116] Peila R, Scordino P, Shanko DB, Caldera F, Trotta F, Ferri A. Synthesis and characterization of β-cyclodextrin nanosponges for N, N-diethyl-meta-toluamide complexation and their application on polyester fabrics. Reactive and Functional Polymers. 2017;**119**:87-94

[117] Zidan MF, Ibrahim HM, Afouna MI, Ibrahim EA. In vitro and in vivo evaluation of cyclodextrin-based nanosponges for enhancing oral bioavailability of atorvastatin calcium. Drug Development and Industrial Pharmacy. 2018;**44**(8):1243-1253

[118] Gabr MM, Mortada SM, Sallam MA. Carboxylate cross-linked cyclodextrin: A nanoporous scaffold for enhancement of rosuvastatin oral bioavailability. European Journal of Pharmaceutical Sciences. 2018;**111**:1-12

[119] Nait Bachir Y, Nait Bachir R, Hadj-Ziane-Zafour A. Nanodispersions stabilized by β-cyclodextrin nanosponges: Application for simultaneous enhancement of bioactivity and stability of sage essential oil. Drug Development and Industrial Pharmacy. 2019;**45**(2):333-347

[120] Mendes C, Meirelles GC, Barp CG, Assreuy J, Silva MA, Ponchel G. Cyclodextrin based nanosponge of norfloxacin: Intestinal permeation enhancement and improved antibacterial activity. Carbohydrate Polymers. 2018;**195**:586-592

[121] Mady FM, Ibrahim M, Ragab S. Cyclodextrin-based nanosponge for improvement of solubility and oral bioavailability of ellagic acid. Pakistan Journal of Pharmaceutical Sciences. 2018;**31**(5):2069-2076

[122] Singh P, Ren X, Guo T, Wu L, Shakya S, He Y, et al. Biofunctionalization of β-cyclodextrin nanosponges using cholesterol. Carbohydrate Polymers. 2018;**190**:23-30

[123] Kumar S, Trotta F, Rao R. Encapsulation of Babchi oil in cyclodextrin-based nanosponges: Physicochemical characterization, photodegradation, and in vitro cytotoxicity studies. Pharmaceutics. 2018;**10**(4):169. DOI: 10.3390/pharmaceutics10040169

[124] Kumar S, Singh KK, Rao R. Enhanced anti-psoriatic efficacy and regulation of oxidative stress of a novel topical babchi oil (*Psoralea corylifolia*) cyclodextrin-based nanogel in a mouse tail model. Journal of Microencapsulation. 2019;**36**(2):140-155. DOI: 10.1080/02652048.2019.1612475

[125] Argenziano M, Haimhoffer A, Bastiancich C, Jicsinszky L, Caldera F, Trotta F, et al. In vitro enhanced skin permeation and retention of imiquimod loaded in β-cyclodextrin nanosponge hydrogel. Pharmaceutics. 2019;**11**(3):138. DOI: 10.3390/pharmaceutics11030138

[126] Loftsson T, Brewster ME. Pharmaceutical applications of cyclodextrins. 1. Drug solubilization and stabilization. Journal of Pharmaceutical Sciences. 1996;**85**(10):1017-1025

[127] Challa R, Ahuja A, Ali J, Khar RK. Cyclodextrins in drug delivery: An updated review. AAPS PharmSciTech. 2005;**6**(2):E329-E357

[128] Harth E, Diaz R. Nanosponge Drug Delivery System More Effective Than Direct Injection. Nanotechnology Now [Internet]. 2010. Available from: https://news.vanderbilt.edu/2010/06/01/nanosponge-drug-delivery-system-more-effective-than-direct-injection-116839/ [Accessed: May 11, 2019]

[129] Adeoye O, Cabral-Marques H. Cyclodextrin nanosystems in oral drug delivery: A mini review. International Journal of Pharmaceutics. 2017;**531**(2):521-531

[130] Healy AM, McDonald BF, Tajber L, Corrigan OI. Characterisation of excipient-free nanoporous microparticles (NPMPs) of bendroflumethiazide. European Journal of Pharmaceutics and Biopharmaceutics. 2008;**69**(3):1182-1186

[131] Nolan LM, Li J, Tajber L, Corrigan OI, Healy AM. Particle engineering of materials for oral inhalation by dry powder inhalers. II—Sodium cromoglicate. International Journal of Pharmaceutics. 2011;**405**(1-2):36-46

[132] Nolan LM, Tajber L, McDonald BF, Barham AS, Corrigan OI, Healy AM. Excipient-free nanoporous microparticles of budesonide for pulmonary delivery. European Journal of Pharmaceutical Sciences. 2009;**37**(5):593-602

[133] Ógáin ON, Li J, Tajber L, Corrigan OI, Healy AM. Particle engineering of materials for oral inhalation by dry powder inhalers. I—Particles of sugar excipients (trehalose and raffinose) for protein delivery. International Journal of Pharmaceutics. 2011;**405**(1-2):23-35

[134] Indira B, Bolisetti SS, Samrat C, Reddy SM, Reddy NS. Nanosponges: A new era in drug delivery. Journal of Pharmacy Research. 2012;**5**(12):5293-5296

Chapter 7

# Effect of Cyclodextrin Derivatization on Solubility and Efficacy of Drugs

*Syed Haroon Khalid, Mehreen Bashir, Sajid Asghar, Tauqeer Hussain Mallhi and Ikram Ullah Khan*

## Abstract

Cyclodextrins (CDs) possess cyclic structure having (α-1,4)-linked glucopyranose units making them less vulnerable to enzymatic degradation as than the linear dextrins. Commonly used natural CDs are α-CD, β-CD, and γ-CD with truncated cone-like appearance having lipophilic central cavity and hydrophilic exterior surface. The problem of low aqueous solubility of natural CDs can be addressed by reacting them with various reagents to produce water-soluble derivatives. CD derivatives can be categorized in many ways depending upon their substituents, biological activity, polarity, and size. The derivatization of natural CDs produces noncrystalline and amorphous forms with higher water solubility that are physically and microbiologically stable for prolonged time period. Variety of methods can be used to determine average degree of substitution for a modified CD. Dissociation by dilution is considered as major release mechanism of drugs from complex. It is essential to optimize the amount of CDs for a given preparation because they can either retard or promote drug delivery through biological membrane.

**Keywords:** natural cyclodextrins, cyclodextrin derivatives, inclusion complex, poorly soluble drugs

## 1. Introduction

Cyclodextrins (CDs), first isolated by Antoine in 1891, are categorized as cyclic oligosaccharides in which glucose units are repeatedly connected through α-1,4-glycosidic linkages. Their unique property is the availability of various hydroxyl groups that serve as active site to form a variety of derivatives and linkages. CDs possess the capability of forming inclusion complexes with various molecules by incorporating them in their inner hydrophobic cavity, which not only alters the biological and physicochemical properties but also expands their magnitude of application [1–3].

Inclusion complexation is basically the formation of hydrogen bonds and Van der Waals' and hydrophobic interactions along with removal of water molecules [4, 5]. CDs are getting popular as food additives, owing to their solubilizing and protecting properties; they can be effectively used for incorporating vitamins, flavors, fragrances, essential oils, and dyes. They not only provide the controlled release of drugs and other incorporated molecules but also mask the obnoxious taste and odor [6–9].

The order of water solubility for commonly used cyclodextrins is as follows: β-CD (18.5 $gL^{-1}$) < α-CD (145$gL^{-1}$) < γ-CD (232 $gL^{-1}$). The crystal state of natural CDs indicates strong molecular bonding (high crystal lattice energy) which in turn results in low aqueous solubility. β-CD has limited application as a solubilizing agent due to its low aqueous solubility, despite low cost, ease of availability, and appropriate cavity size. The most likely justification of lower solubility of β-CD is inadequate hydration by water molecule due to intramolecular hydrogen bond interaction offered by optimally arranged secondary hydroxyl groups [10]. Another possible elucidation of low aqueous solubility is the formation of aggregates that leads to unfavorable interactions with the hydrogen bonded structure of water molecule as proposed by Colman and coworkers [11]. β-CD shows Bs-type behavior in phase solubility graph when added to the aqueous drug solution or suspension due to precipitation of respective CD inclusion complex.

The solubilizing power of parent CDs can be enhanced by adopting many different strategies, but the most interesting of them is the derivatization of CDs. The hydroxyl groups of CDs can be substituted to yield a variety of derivatives with significantly high aqueous solubility [12–14]. This chapter discusses the various strategies to functionalize the CDs and the resultant improvement in the aqueous solubility of formed complexes.

## 2. Functionalized CDs

Parent CDs can be modified through structural modifications by incorporating hydrophilic moieties that will ultimately result in significant increase in aqueous solubility. Furthermore, the inclusion complexes formed by modified CDs have higher complexation efficiencies than that of parent CDs. Rekharsky and Inoue reported various examples of thermodynamic parameters of inclusion complexes involving derivatized CDs [5].

It is noteworthy that derivatization of CDs does not always enhance the complexation. The inhibition and promotion of complexation solely depends upon the type of substituents. Although the strong electrostatic force of attraction between the cationic substituents and organic anion was predicted to promote complexation, paradoxical effect was observed when the complexation of 2-naphthalene sulfonate was reduced with polyamine derivatives of β-CD. An unfavorable entropic effect may be involved that results in decrease in complexation [15]. On the other hand, a favorable electrostatic interaction occurs that leads to formation of zwitterionic corona by substituting both cationic and anionic groups at the primary face that will ultimately enhance the complexation of amino acids [16].

The interdependence of numerous molecular parameters including type of substituent at the CDs, contribution of hydrophobic, and charge character of the guest moiety and competitive self-complexation (possible inclusion complexation of substituent moiety inside the core of CD) was discussed in detail by Kean and his coworkers [17]. While dealing with ionic species, electrostatic effects are usually dominated which exert a paradoxical effect. Based on this status quo, the inclusion complexation of charged CD with organic ions must be evaluated on the basis of electrostatic interactions. The properties of modified CDs are governed by the location of hydroxyl groups on the parent CDs that are going to be substituted. Three different hydroxyl groups that exert different reactivities are located on the glucose repeating unit of a CD molecule, including one primary hydroxyl group attached to

C6 (at the narrow side) and two secondary hydroxyl groups attached to C2 and C3 (at wider side).

Most common derivatives of CDs are discussed in this section.

### 2.1 Methyl derivatives of CDs

There is variety of ways to perform methylation of native cyclodextrins:

Formerly methyl derivatives were synthesized by using either methyl iodide or dimethyl sulfate [18]. These two reagents are highly toxic and unsafe so may be detrimental to the environment as well as human being. Based on this status quo, it is mandatory to seek new and novel synthetic method to replace these toxic chemicals.

Dimethyl carbonate being eco-friendly could be an attractive alternate in this scenario [19]. The synthesis involves addition of β-CD in dimethylformamide solution followed by stirring until clear solution is obtained. Potassium carbonate is added as catalyst followed by dropwise addition of dimethyl carbonate, and mixture is allowed to stir for the next 48 hours. The catalyst and dimethyl carbonate are removed to produce syrupy consistency. At the end, this concentrate is treated with acetone followed by its removal by filtration. Finally, the product is treated with ether two to three times, and after filtration white powdered product is obtained as indicated in **Figure 1**.

An important feature of methyl β-CD is its degree of substitution that has marked effect on drug solubilization, so it must be carefully investigated [20]. **Table 1** gives the use of methyl derivatives of β-CD with effect on solubility and efficacy of various drugs.

This pharmaceutically significant methylated derivative of β-CD has the following advantages:

- Easy availability (as dry powder/aqueous solution 50%)
- Good water solubility
- Cost-effective
- High inclusion capacity for hydrophobic drugs

### 2.2 Hydroxypropyl CDs

The replacement of hydroxyl groups of CD by 2-hydroxypropyl moiety can be done by the reaction of CD with propylene oxide in an alkaline aqueous solution (**Figure 2a**) [31]. An isopropylene (oligomeric hydroxypropylene) side chain is formed for high degree of substitution (**Figure 2b**).

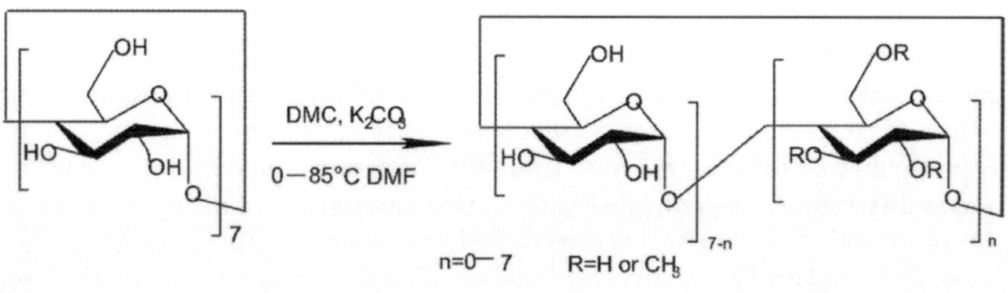


**Figure 1.**
*Synthesis of methyl β-CD [21].*

| Author | Drug | Additives (if used) | Effects |
|---|---|---|---|
| Schipper et al. [22] | Insulin | — | Improved nasal absorption |
| Schipper et al. [23] | Salmon calcitonin | — | Enhanced nasal penetration |
| Sigurdsson et al. [24] | Dexamethasone | — | Localized drug delivery to anterior eye segment |
| Soares-Sobrinho et al. [25] | Benznidazole | PVP, HPMC | Enhanced solubility, reduced toxicity |
| Mathiron et al. [26] | Midazolam | — | Improved solubility, protective effect on drug degradation |
| Chao et al. [27] | Ofloxacin | — | Significant increase in solubility, improved pharmacological efficacy |
| Vieira et al. [28] | Efavirenz | PVP | Improved dissolution profile, increased stability |
| Rassu et al. [29] | Deferoxamine mesylate | — | Improved bioavailability, avoidance of systemic exposure |
| Terauchi et al. [30] | Simvastatin | — | Improved solubility, effective bone regeneration therapy |

**Table 1.**
*Effect of methyl derivatives of β-CD on solubility and efficacy of drugs.*

The characterization of finally synthesized hydroxypropyl derivatives involves determination of average number of substituents on the cyclodextrin molecule (degree of substitution). According to latest US and European pharmacopoeias, the acceptable range for DS is 2.8–10.5 for HPβCD. Degree of substitution can be measured by a variety of techniques including near-infrared reflectance spectroscopy, nuclear magnetic resonance (NMR), microcalorimetric titration [33], mass spectrometry (MS), differential scanning calorimetry (DSC) [34], and reductive-cleavage and methylation analysis.

Encapsin™ and Molecusol™ are the trade names of commercially available form of hydroxyalkyl derivative (2-hydroxypropyl-β-CD). Various clinical trials have been performed with this derivative besides its use in technological, toxicological, and pharmaceutical experiments [35]. Being the most thoroughly studied derivative, FDA has approved Sporanox™ by Janssen using the same derivatives as molecular carrier. The hydroxypropyl derivative of β-CD and γ-CD have been widely used for solubility enhancement and leading to increase in efficacy of various drugs as illustrated in **Tables 2** and **3**.

## 2.3 Sulfoalkylated CDs

Almost more than 180 articles had focused on the preparation and use of charged (anionic) CD derivatives by the end of July 1998.The glucopyranose unit present in the native CD ring could be directly substituted with charged moiety, or a neutral spacer group may be used for the insertion [49]. Such functional groups can be inserted at different degrees of substitution (DS) and have variable sizes, so the final product of modified CD derivative may be influenced by electronic and steric factors.

The sulfopropyl and sulfobutyl derivatives of beta-CDs are produced by reacting native CD with propane sultone and butane sultone, respectively, in an alkaline aqueous solution as shown in **Figure 3**.

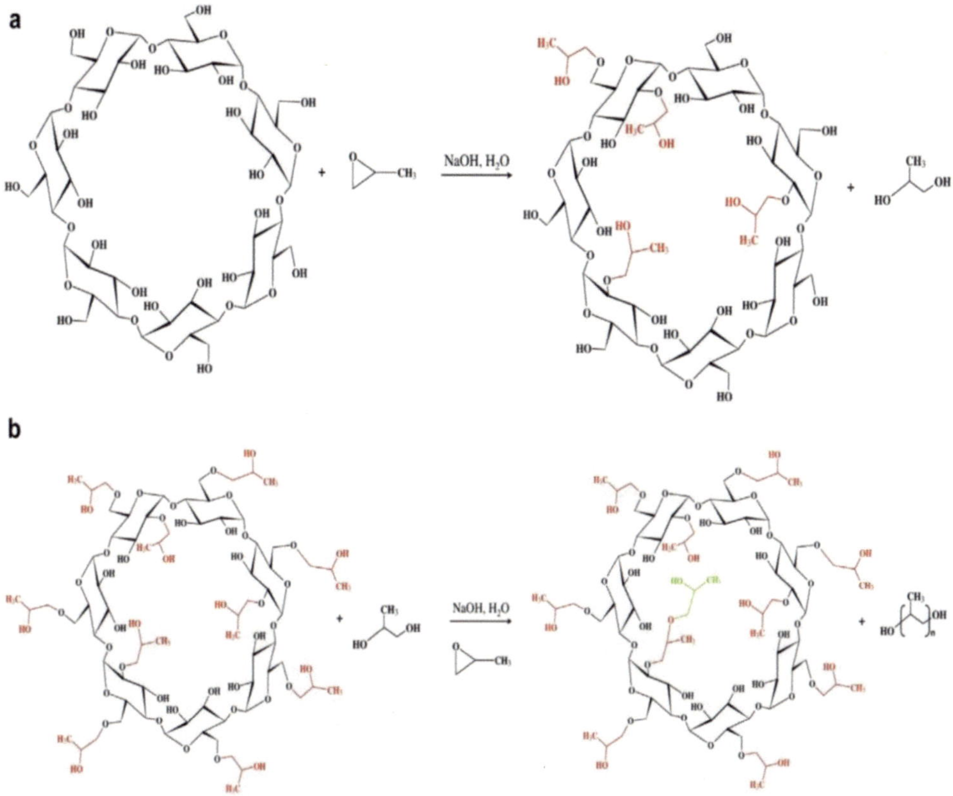

**Figure 2.**
*Reaction scheme for HPβCD synthesis: (a) low DS, (b) high DS [32].*

| Author | Drug | Other additives (if present) | Effects |
|---|---|---|---|
| Kaur et al. 2004 [36] | Acetazolamide | PVA, PVP, HPMC, Carbopol 940 | Improved solubility, effective drug permeation, improved corneal transport |
| Chowdary et al. [37] | Celecoxib | PVP, HPMC, PEG | Improved solubility, higher CE by ternary complexation |
| El-Maradny et al. [38] | Meloxicam | PVP, L-ARG | Improved solubility, quick pain relieving effect, faster drug release with ternary complex |
| Manali Shah et al. [39] | Etoricoxib | PVP, L-ARG | Enhanced dissolution profile, improved oral bioavailability |
| Asbahr et al. [40] | Finasteride | PVP, chitosan | Positive effect on drug solubility, inc. in bulk of formulation so can be used in solid dosage forms |
| Mummidi and Jayanthi [41] | Isradipine | PVP, HPMC, PEG | Marked increase in solubilizing efficiency, improved dissolution with ternary complexes |
| Pacheco et al. [42] | Albendazole | PVA | Enhanced solubility, improved intrinsic dissolution rate |
| Jadhav and Pore [43] | Bosentan | Arginine (ARG) | Enhanced solubility and dissolution profile |

**Table 2.**
*Effects of HPβCD on solubility and efficacy of drugs.*

| Author | Drug | Other additives (if present) | Effects |
|---|---|---|---|
| Zhou et al. [44] | Baicalein | — | Higher drug absorption, better stability, enhanced release profile |
| Soica et al. [45] | Oleanolic acid, ursolic acid | — | Enhanced aqueous solubility, marked antiproliferative activity |
| Misiuk and Jasiuk 2014 [46] | Bupropion | — | Improved release, rapid absorption, enhanced encapsulation efficiency |
| Misiuk et al. [47] | Ceftazidime | — | Improved aqueous solubility, improved stability as suggested by NMR study |
| Wathoni et al. [48] | Curcumin | — | Increased solubility, enhanced antioxidant activity |

**Table 3.**
*Effects of HPγCD on solubility and efficacy of drugs.*

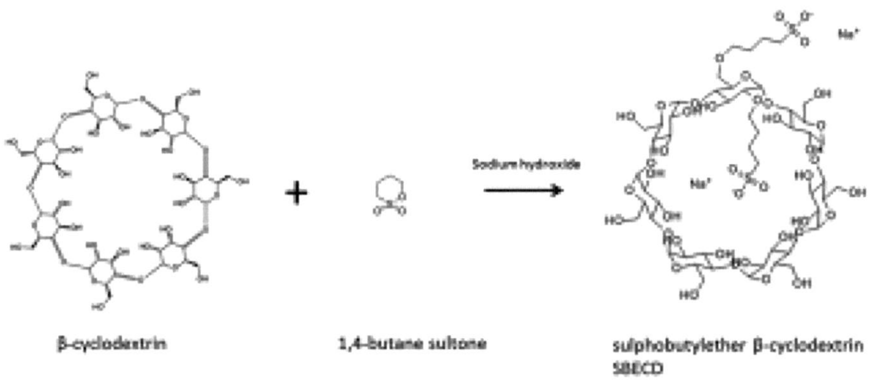


**Figure 3.**
*Synthesis of SBE-β-CD [50].*

Sulfobutylated β-CD with seven substituents is considered as suitable derivative and is commercially available under the trade name of Captisol™ by CyDex. Resveratrol is complexed with sulfobutylether derivatives of β-CD and increased the anticancer activity with increase in solubility of resveratrol as well [51].

## 2.4 Sulfated CDs

A class of water-soluble CD derivatives having anti-angiogenic, biological, and anticancer properties is sulfated CDs. As the tumor growth is dependent on angiogenesis, the use of these derivatives could be a unique approach for the treatment of solid tumors, as reported by Folkman et al. in early 1970 [52]. In addition to these properties, they also possess antilipemic, antiviral, and anti-inflammatory effects [53].

Reaction of CD in absolute dimethylformamide with pyridine sulfur trioxide gives better yield of sulfated derivatives of CDs [54]. Besides their use as solubility enhancers, these derivatives also provide protection against gentamicin-induced nephrotoxicity and have no hemolytic properties, so can be effectively used in clinical studies [55]. **Figure 4** presents the scheme of preparation of sulfated β-CD.

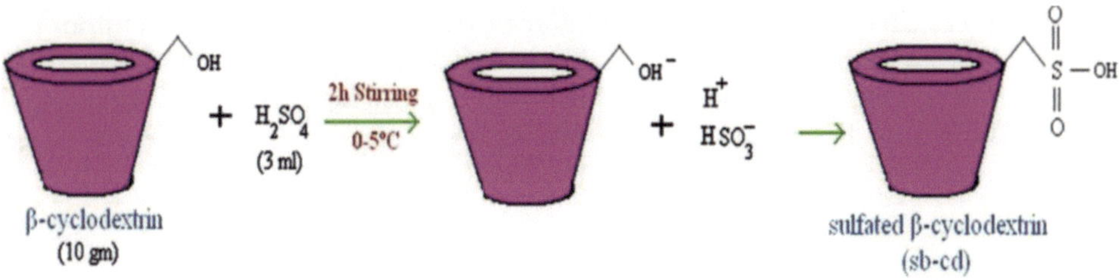


**Figure 4.**
*Synthesis of sulfated β-CD [56].*

### 2.5 Guidelines regarding synthesis of CD derivatives

The following guidelines should be strictly followed during the synthesis of CD derivatives in order to get the better solubility and complexing ability:

- Although the substituents at primary hydroxyl side may influence other uses, they do not exert much effect on the complexation. The pH of the medium is decisive that either the secondary hydroxyl side or primary side will be substituted. Moderately basic medium will favor secondary hydroxyl substitution, whereas primary hydroxyl side will get substituted in strong basic medium [57].

- To avoid the deformation of cavity shape, avoid the bulky substitution which may crowd each other. Although the CD torus is made of anhydroglucose repeating units which are quite rigid, they are connected to each other through single glycosidic bonds. As torus is stabilized by hydrogen bonds between the secondary hydroxyls on adjacent glucose unit, the stabilizing effect of hydrogen bonding is diminished by secondary hydroxyl substitution. Finally, the anhydroglucose units may tilt out the defined torus shape due to introduction of steric strain between substituting units present on the adjacent anhydroglucose residues [35].

- The water-soluble CDs are used either in solid form or in concentrated solution state. Some substituting groups have the tendency to incorporate in the core of CDs, so they compete with active drug molecules for inclusion complexation. Therefore, it is mandatory to select those substituents that are unable to fit in the cavity of CDs [58].

- A glucopyranose unit of cyclodextrin ring contains how many substituted hydroxyl groups are defined as its degree of substitution. One mole of glucopyranose unit contains three reactive hydroxyl groups so the maximum possible numbers of substituents are 18, 21, and 24 for α-, β-, and γ- CDs, respectively. Controlling the degree of substitution is important in producing the desired properties in functionalized CDs.

## 3. Conclusion

Using different functional groups, modified CDs could play a pivotal role in improving limited drug stability and boosting aqueous solubility and dissolution behavior of drugs with poor water solubility. In order to use full potential of CDs as a drug delivery carrier, the nature and degree of functionalization play an important role. However, the future research should focus on the use of green chemistry for CDs' functionalization, and the attention should also be paid to the toxicokinetic profiling of the modified CDs to establish their safety and efficacy at the same time.

## Conflict of interest

There is no conflict of interest among the listed authors.

## Author details

Syed Haroon Khalid[1*], Mehreen Bashir[1], Sajid Asghar[1], Tauqeer Hussain Mallhi[2] and Ikram Ullah Khan[1]

1 Department of Pharmaceutics, Faculty of Pharmaceutical Sciences, Government College University, Faisalabad, Pakistan

2 Department of Clinical Pharmacy, Jouf University, Sakaka, Kingdom of Saudi Arabia

*Address all correspondence to: haroonkhalid80@gmail.com and syedharoonkhalid@gcuf.edu.pk

## References

[1] Kurkov SV, Loftsson T. Cyclodextrins. International Journal of Pharmaceutics. 2013;**453**:167-180. DOI: 10.1016/j.ijpharm.2012.06.055

[2] Brewster ME, Loftsson T. Cyclodextrins as pharmaceutical solubilizers. Advanced Drug Delivery Reviews. 2007;**59**:645-666. DOI: 10.1016/j.addr.2007.05.012

[3] Del Valle EM. Cyclodextrins and their uses: A review. Process Biochemistry. 2004;**39**:1033-1046. DOI: 10.1016/S0032-9592(03)00258-9

[4] Acuña-Rougier C, Olea-Azar C. Thermodynamic and geometric study of diasteroisomeric complexes formed by racemic flavanones and three cyclodextrins through NMR. Journal of Inclusion Phenomena and Macrocyclic Chemistry. 2013;**75**:119-136. DOI: 10.1007/s10847-012-0153-5

[5] Rekharsky MV, Inoue Y. Complexation thermodynamics of cyclodextrins. Chemical Reviews. 1998;**98**:1875-1918. DOI: 10.1021/cr970015o

[6] Astray G, Gonzalez-Barreiro C, MejutoJC,Rial-OteroR,Simal-GandaraJ. A review on the use of cyclodextrins in foods. Food Hydrocolloids. 2009;**23**:1631-1640. DOI: 10.1016/j.foodhyd.2009.01.001

[7] Szente L, Szejtli J. Cyclodextrins as food ingredients. Trends in Food Science and Technology. 2004;**15**:137-142. DOI: 10.1016/j.tifs.2003.09.019

[8] Szejtli J, Szente L. Elimination of bitter, disgusting tastes of drugs and foods by cyclodextrins. European Journal of Pharmaceutics and Biopharmaceutics. 2005;**61**:115-125. DOI: 10.1016/j.ejpb.2005.05.006

[9] Loftsson T, Brewster ME, Masson M. Role of cyclodextrins in improving oral drug delivery. American Journal of Drug Delivery. 2004;**2**:261-275. DOI: 10.2165/00137696-200402040-00006

[10] Miyazawa I, Ueda H, Nagase H, Endo T, Kobayashi S, Nagai T. Physicochemical properties and inclusion complex formation of δ-cyclodextrin. European Journal of Pharmaceutical Sciences. 1995;**3**:153-162. DOI: 10.1016/0928-0987(95)00006-Y

[11] Coleman AW, Nicolis I, Keller N, Dalbiez JP. Aggregation of cyclodextrins: An explanation of the abnormal solubility of β-cyclodextrin. Journal of Inclusion Phenomena and Molecular Recognition in Chemistry. 1992;**13**:139-143. DOI: 10.1007/BF01053637

[12] Szejtli J. The properties and potential uses of cyclodextrin derivatives. Journal of Inclusion Phenomena and Molecular Recognition in Chemistry. 1992;**14**:25-36. DOI: 10.1007/BF01041363

[13] Uekama K. Pharmaceutical uses of cyclodextrin derivatives. In: High Performance Biomaterials. A Comprehensive Guide to Medical and Pharmaceutical Applications. Szycher M, editor. Technomic: Lancaster, PA; 1991. pp. 789-806

[14] Szejtli J. Introduction and general overview of cyclodextrin chemistry. Chemical Reviews. 1998;**98**:1743-1754. DOI: 10.1021/cr970022c

[15] Inoue Y, Liu Y, Tong LH, Shen BJ, Jin DS. Calorimetric titration of inclusion complexation with modified. Beta.-cyclodextrins. Enthalpy-entropy compensation in host-guest complexation: From ionophore to cyclodextrin and cyclophane. Journal of the American Chemical Society. 1993;**115**:10637-10644. DOI: 10.1021/ja00076a023

[16] Tabushi I, Kuroda Y, Mizutani T. Artificial receptors for amino acids in water. Local environmental effect on polar recognition by 6A-amino-6B-carboxy- and 6B-amino-6A-carboxy-. Beta.-cyclodextrins. Journal of the American Chemical Society. 1986;**108**:4514-4518. DOI: 10.1021/ja00275a043

[17] Kean SD, May BL, Clements P, Lincoln SF, Easton CJH. Host–guest complexation of aromatic carboxylic acids and their conjugate bases by 6 A-(ω-aminoalkylamino)-6 A-deoxy-β-cyclodextrins† in aqueous solution. Journal of the Chemical Society, Perkin Transactions. 1999;**2**:1257-1264. DOI: 10.1039/A806488A

[18] Yuan LM. Effect of mobile phase additive on chiral separation. Separation and Purification Technology. 2008;**63**:701-705. DOI: 10.1016/j.seppur.2008.06.021

[19] Tundo P, Selva M. The chemistry of dimethyl carbonate. Accounts of Chemical Research. 2002;**35**:706-716. DOI: 10.1021/ar010076f

[20] Gan Y, Zhang Y, Xiao C, Zhou C, Zhao Y. A novel preparation of methyl-β-cyclodextrin from dimethyl carbonate and β-cyclodextrin. Carbohydrate Research. 2011;**346**:389-392. DOI: 10.1016/j.carres.2010.05.028

[21] Available from: http://www.google.com/search?biw=1366&bih=576&tbm=isch&sa=1&ei=PgvvXICpLZHFwQKJgK-YAQ&q=synthesis+of+methyl+%CE%B2-Cyclodextrin&oq=synthesis+of+methyl+%CE%B2-Cyclodextrin&gs 1=img.3...165667.172378..178711...0.0..0.358.2515.0jij5j3......0....1j2..gws-wiz-img.......0j0i67.kdloQir1DqM#imgrc=qywHXUGYUQO96M:

[22] Schipper NG, Romeijn SG, Verhoef JC, Merkus FW. Nasal insulin delivery with dimethyl-β-cyclodextrin as an absorption enhancer in rabbits: Powder more effective than liquid formulations. Pharmaceutical Research. 1993;**10**:682-686. DOI: 10.1023/A:1018999414088

[23] Schipper NG, Verhoef JC, Romeijn SG, Merkus FW. Methylated β-cyclodextrins are able to improve the nasal absorption of salmon calcitonin. Calcified Tissue International. 1995;**56**:280-282. DOI: 10.1007/BF00318047

[24] Sigurdsson HH, Konráðsdóttir F, Loftsson T, Stefansson E. Topical and systemic absorption in delivery of dexamethasone to the anterior and posterior segments of the eye. Acta Ophthalmologica Scandinavica. 2007;**85**:598-602. DOI: 10.1111/j.1600-0420.2007.00885.x

[25] Soares-Sobrinho JL, Santos FL, Lyra MA, Alves LD, Rolim LA, Lima AA, et al. Benznidazole drug delivery by binary and multicomponent inclusion complexes using cyclodextrins and polymers. Carbohydrate Polymers. 2012;**89**:323-330. DOI: 10.1016/j.carbpol.2012.02.042

[26] Mathiron D, Marçon F, Dubaele JM, Cailleu D, Pilard S, Djedaïni-pilard F. Benefits of methylated cyclodextrins in the development of midazolam pharmaceutical formulations. Journal of Pharmaceutical Sciences. 2013;**102**:2102-2111. DOI: 10.1002/jps.23558

[27] Chao J, Liu Y, Zhang Y, Zhang J, Zhang Y, Guo Z, et al. Investigation of the inclusion behavior of ofloxacin with methyl-β-cyclodextrin. Journal of Molecular Liquids. 2014;**200**:404-409. DOI: 10.1016/j.molliq.2014.11.015

[28] Vieira AC, Fontes DA, Chaves LL, Alves LD, de Freitas Neto JL, Soares MF, et al. Multicomponent systems with cyclodextrins and hydrophilic polymers for the delivery of Efavirenz. Carbohydrate Polymers. 2015;**130**:133-140. DOI: 10.1016/j.carbpol.2015.04.050

[29] Rassu G, Soddu E, Cossu M, Brundu A, Cerri G, Marchetti N, et al. Solid microparticles based on chitosan or methyl-β-cyclodextrin: A first formulative approach to increase the nose-to-brain transport of deferoxamine mesylate. Journal of Controlled Release. 2015;**201**:68-77. DOI: 10.1016/j.jconrel.2015.01.025

[30] Terauchi M, Inada T, Tonegawa A, Tamura A, Yamaguchi S, Harada K, et al. Supramolecular inclusion complexation of simvastatin with methylated β-cyclodextrins for promoting osteogenic differentiation. International Journal of Biological Macromolecules. 2016;**93**:1492-1498. DOI: 10.1016/j.ijbiomac.2016.01.114

[31] Pitha J, Szabo L, Fales HM. Reaction of cyclodextrins with propylene oxide or with glycidol: Analysis of product distribution. Carbohydrate Research. 1987;**168**:191-198. DOI: 10.1016/0008-6215(87)80025-3

[32] Available from: http://www.google.com/search?q=Reaction+scheme+for+HPBCD+synthesis&source=Inms&tbm=isch&sa=X&ved=oahUKEwiY-Lj 6cHiAhXBoKQKHdfkBGkQAUIDigB&biw=1366&bih=576#imgrc=fwlmslwWc6M3DM:

[33] Reer O, Müller BW. Determination of the degree of substitution of chemically modified cyclodextrins by a microcalorimetric titration technique. International Journal of Pharmaceutics. 1994;**104**:239-246. DOI: 10.1016/0378-5173(94)90164-3

[34] Novák C, Pokol G, Sztatisz J, Szente L, Szejtli J. Determination of the degree of substitution of hydroxypropylated β-cyclodextrins by differential scanning calorimetry. Analytica Chimica Acta. 1993;**282**:313-316. DOI: 10.1016/0003-2670(93)80216-8

[35] Szente L, Szejtli J. Highly soluble cyclodextrin derivatives: Chemistry, properties, and trends in development. Advanced Drug Delivery Reviews. 1999;**36**:17-28. DOI: 10.1016/S0169-409X(98)00092-1

[36] Kaur IP, Kapil M, Smitha R, Aggarwal D. Development of topically effective formulations of acetazolamide using HP-β-CD-polymer co-complexes. Current Drug Delivery. 2004;**1**:65-72. DOI: 10.2174/1567201043480054

[37] Chowdary KP, Srinivas SV. Influence of hydrophilic polymers on celecoxib complexation with hydroxypropyl β-cyclodextrin. AAPS PharmSciTech. 2006;**7**:E184-E189. DOI: 10.1208/pt070

[38] El-Maradny H, Mortada S, Kamel O, Hikal A. Characterization of ternary complexes of meloxicam-HPβCD and PVP or L-arginine prepared by the spray-drying technique. Acta Pharmaceutica. 2008;**58**:455-466. DOI: 10.2478/v10007-008-0029-9

[39] Shah M, Karekar P, Sancheti P, Vyas V, Pore Y. Effect of PVP K30 and/or L-arginine on stability constant of etoricoxib–HPβCD inclusion complex: Preparation and characterization of etoricoxib–HPβCD binary system. Drug Development and Industrial Pharmacy. 2009;**35**:118-129. DOI: 10.1080/03639040802220292

[40] Asbahr AC, Franco L, Barison A, Silva CW, Ferraz HG, Rodrigues LN. Binary and ternary inclusion complexes of finasteride in HPβCD and polymers: Preparation and characterization. Bioorganic & Medicinal Chemistry. 2009;**17**:2718-2723. DOI: 10.1016/j.bmc.2009.02.044

[41] Mummidi V, Jayanthi V. Effect of hydrophilic polymers on isradipine complexation with hydroxypropyl β-cyclodextrin. Drug Development and Industrial Pharmacy. 2013;**39**:970-977. DOI: 10.3109/03639045.2012.686508

[42] Pacheco PA, Rodrigues LN, Ferreira JF, Gomes AC, Veríssimo CJ, Louvandini H, et al. Inclusion complex and nanoclusters of cyclodextrin to increase the solubility and efficacy of albendazole. Parasitology Research. 2018;**117**:705-712. DOI: 10.1007/s0043

[43] Jadhav P, Pore Y. Physicochemical, thermodynamic and analytical studies on binary and ternary inclusion complexes of bosentan with hydroxypropyl-β-cyclodextrin. Bulletin of Faculty of Pharmacy, Cairo University. 2017;**55**:147-154. DOI: 10.1016/j.bfopcu.2016.12.004

[44] Zhou Q, Zhong L, Wei X, Dou W, Chou G, Wang Z. Baicalein and hydroxypropyl-γ-cyclodextrin complex in poloxamer thermal sensitive hydrogel for vaginal administration. International Journal of Pharmaceutics. 2013;**454**:125-134. DOI: 10.1016/j.ijpharm.2013.07.006

[45] Soica C, Oprean C, Borcan F, Danciu C, Trandafirescu C, Coricovac D, et al. The synergistic biologic activity of oleanolic and ursolic acids in complex with hydroxypropyl-γ-cyclodextrin. Molecules. 2014;**19**:4924-4940. DOI: 10.3390/molecules19044924

[46] Misiuk W, Jasiuk E. Study of the inclusion interaction of HP-γ-cyclodextrin with bupropion and its analytical application. Journal of Molecular Structure. 2014;**1060**:272-279. DOI: 10.1016/j.molstruc.2013.12.056

[47] Misiuk W. Investigation of inclusion complex of HP-γ-cyclodextrin with ceftazidime. Journal of Molecular Liquids. 2016;**224**:387-392. DOI: 10.1016/j.molliq.2016.10.009

[48] Wathoni N, Motoyama K, Higashi T, Okajima M, Kaneko T, Arima H. Enhancement of curcumin wound healing ability by complexation with 2-hydroxypropyl-γ-cyclodextrin in sacran hydrogel film. International Journal of Biological Macromolecules. 2017;**98**:268-276. DOI: 10.1016/j.ijbiomac.2017.01.144

[49] Rajewski RA. Development and evaluation of the usefulness and parenteral safety of modified cyclodextrins. 5332-5332. Order No. DA9110909 from: Diss Abstr Int B; 1991

[50] Available from: http://www.google.com/search?q=synthesis+of+SBE-%CE%B2-CD&source=lnms&tbm=isch&sa=X&ved=oahUKEwjWytO6sHiAhVFr6QKHYXyDXoQAUIDigB&biw=1366&bih=576#imgrc=gsB7mNy3Gv4-EM:

[51] Venuti V, Cannavà C, Cristiano MC, Fresta M, Majolino D, Paolino D, et al. A characterization study of resveratrol/sulfobutyl ether-β-cyclodextrin inclusion complex and in vitro anticancer activity. Colloids and Surfaces. B, Biointerfaces. 2014;**115**:22-28. DOI: 10.1016/j.colsurfb.2013.11.025

[52] Folkman J, Weisz PB, Joullie MM, Li WW, Ewing WR. Control of angiogenesis with synthetic heparin substitutes. Science. 1989;**243**:1490-1493. DOI: 10.1126/science.2467380

[53] Anand R, Nayyar S, Pitha J, Merril CR. Sulphated sugar alpha-cyclodextrin sulphate, a uniquely potent anti-HIV agent, also exhibits marked synergism with AZT, and lymphoproliferative activity. Antiviral Chemistry and Chemotherapy. 1990;**1**:41-46. DOI: 10.1177/095632029000100107

[54] Pitha J, Mallis LM, Lamb DJ, Irie T, Uekama K. Cyclodextrin sulfates: Characterization as polydisperse and amorphous mixtures. Pharmaceutical Research. 1991;**8**:1151-1154. DOI: 10.1023/A:1015854402122

[55] Shiotani K, Irie T, Uekama K, Ishimaru Y. Cyclodextrin sulfates in parenteral use: Protection against gentamicin nephrotoxicity in the rat. European Journal of Pharmaceutical

Sciences. 1995;**3**:139-151. DOI: 10.1016/0928-0987(95)00008

[56] Available from: http://www.google.com/search?biw=1366&bih=576&tbm=isch&sa=1&ei=DA7vXI3jAcPUsAfFxbqwDw&q=synthesis+of+sulfated+beta+Cyclodextrin&oq=synthesis+of+sulfated+beta+Cyclodextrin&gs1=img.3...98943.106317..106999...o.o..o.287.2376.oj5j6......o....1j2..gws-img.......35i39jo.-K9CA2MG-vc#imgrc=HuSGnVpvSKSLsM:

[57] Pitha J, Rao CT, Lindberg B, Seffers P. Distribution of substituents in 2-hydroxypropyl ethers of cyclomaltoheptaose. Carbohydrate Research. 1990;**200**:429-435. DOI: 10.1016/0008-6215(90)84208-C

[58] Harata K, Rao CT, Pitha J, Fukunaga K, Uekama K. Crystal structure of 2-O-[(S)-2-hydroxypropyl] cyclomaltoheptaose. Carbohydrate Research. 1991;**222**:37-45. DOI: 10.1016/0008-6215(91)89004-Y